# Veterinary Euthanasia Techniques

## A Practical Guide

# Veterinary Euthanasia Techniques

## A Practical Guide

Kathleen  A. Cooney, DVM, MS

Jolynn R. Chappell, DVM

Robert J. Callan, DVM, MS

Bruce A. Connally, DVM, MS

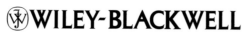
WILEY-BLACKWELL

A John Wiley & Sons, Ltd., Publication

This edition first published 2012 © 2012 by John Wiley & Sons, Inc.

Wiley-Blackwell is an imprint of John Wiley & Sons, formed by the merger of Wiley's global Scientific, Technical and Medical business with Blackwell Publishing.

*Editorial offices:*   2121 State Avenue, Ames, Iowa 50014-8300, USA
                      The Atrium, Southern Gate, Chichester, West Sussex, PO19 8SQ, UK
                      9600 Garsington Road, Oxford, OX4 2DQ, UK

For details of our global editorial offices, for customer services and for information about how to apply for permission to reuse the copyright material in this book please see our website at www.wiley.com/wiley-blackwell.

*Library of Congress Cataloging-in-Publication Data*

Veterinary euthanasia techniques : a practical guide / Robert Callan ... [et al.].
       p. ; cm.
   Includes bibliographical references and index.
   ISBN 978-0-470-95918-3 (pbk. : alk. paper)
   1. Euthanasia of animals–Technique–Handbooks, manuals, etc.   2. Veterinary anesthesia–Handbooks, manuals, etc.   I. Callan, Robert J.
   [DNLM: 1. Euthanasia, Animal–methods.   2. Animals, Domestic.   SF 756.394]
   SF756.394.V48 2012
   636.089′796–dc23

                                                            2011052835

A catalogue record for this book is available from the British Library.

Wiley also publishes its books in a variety of electronic formats. Some content that appears in print may not be available in electronic books.

Set in 9/12.5 pt Interstate Light by Aptara® Inc., New Delhi, India
Printed and bound in Malaysia by Vivar Printing Sdn Bhd

**Disclaimer**

1  2012

# Contents

# About the Authors

**Dr. Kathleen A. Cooney** is the founder and owner of Home to Heaven, PC, a euthanasia specialty service based in northern Colorado. Since 2006, Dr. Cooney has helped thousands of pets pass peacefully in the comfort of their homes. Dr. Cooney graduated from Colorado State University's (CSU) DVM program in 2004. She is a strong advocate for education and teaches in-home euthanasia techniques, along with client communication, to junior veterinary students in CSU's veterinary medical program. Dr. Cooney has developed numerous webinars and continuing-education opportunities for veterinarians regarding the many facets of companion-animal euthanasia and hospice care. She also created an online national pet euthanasia directory and operates the nation's first pet euthanasia center in Loveland, CO. Her first book, *In-home Pet Euthanasia Techniques*, was completed in 2011 and can be found as an eBook. Dr. Cooney is an active member of the International Association for Animal Hospice and Palliative Care (IAAHPC) presenting talks on end-of-life care. She was also a member of the companion animal working group for the 2011 American Veterinary Medical Association (AVMA) Euthanasia Panel proceedings and received the Rising Star Veterinarian Award from the Colorado Veterinary Medical Association later that year.

**Dr. Jolynn R. Chappell** graduated from Colorado State University College of Veterinary Medicine in 1991. In 1992, she opened Aspen Wing Bird and Animal Hospital in Loveland, CO. Her clinic specializes in exotic medicine and works to maintain the highest level of care. For years, Dr. Chappell taught avian husbandry to CSU students; she is certified in medical acupuncture with an emphasis in avian medicine, and is an active member of numerous exotic-based associations. She is a respected member among Colorado's exotic practitioners and receives referrals throughout Colorado, Nebraska, and Wyoming. Her professional interests include anything pertaining to exotic medicine as well as wildlife work with the Colorado Division of Wildlife.

**Dr. Robert J. Callan** is a professor at Colorado State University in the Department of Clinical Sciences and service head of the Livestock Medicine and Surgery Service at the CSU James L. Voss Veterinary Teaching Hospital. He obtained his DVM degree at Oregon State University in 1986 and then obtained an MS in reproductive physiology at Utah State University in 1988. Dr. Callan completed a residency in large animal internal medicine at the University of Wisconsin-Madison where he also obtained a PhD in virology in 1996. He has been a faculty member at CSU since 1996 and provides clinical care for ruminant and camelid livestock. Dr. Callan is a member of the American College of Veterinary Internal Medicine. His research interests focus on infectious diseases and immunity in livestock.

**Dr. Bruce A. Connally** graduated from Colorado State University College of Veterinary Medicine in 1979 and joined a primarily large animal practice in Lander, WY. He purchased that practice 3 years later, and purchased another in Riverton, WY, in 1987. A series of injuries forced Dr. Connally to sell these practices and become a technical services veterinarian for SmithKline Beecham in 1989. A year later, he became a field service veterinarian for Michigan State University where he treated horses and camelids. He also completed a Master's degree in Large Animal Clinical Sciences at MSU in 1993. In 1998, Dr. Connally returned to Wyoming and established Wyoming Equine, an ambulatory practice for horses. In 2004, he joined the equine ambulatory service at Colorado State University. Up until the summer of 2011, Dr. Connally was an assistant professor at CSU and the senior faculty member in the equine ambulatory service. He is currently practicing equine medicine in Wyoming.

# Acknowledgments

**W**e the authors would like to thank all those within the veterinary and scientific community who have helped to pioneer the techniques discussed in this book. It is through their dedication to medicine and the betterment of animal care that techniques like these exist today. We recognize the hours of work, years of study, and ever-present compassion that has gone into this body of knowledge. Our hope is that everyone reading will approve of our collaborative effort here. Writing this book gave us the opportunity to reflect on our own perceptions of euthanasia and our commitment to a "good death."

No project such as this book is accomplished without mentoring, guidance, help, and support from others. A special thank you to those people in our immediate world that provided guidance and/or who have shared their own successes and challenges with euthanasia: Doug Fakkema, Jan Shearer, Celeste Guerrero, Sheila McGuirk, Sue Semrad, Paul Lunn, Benjamin Darien, Maryann McCrackin, Gene Komer, John MacNeil, Jessica Pierce, Heather Craig, Lesya Ukrainchuk, Tim Holt, Stacey Byers, Dave Van Metre, Frank Garry, and Page Dinsmore. Another special acknowledgment to Michele Graham for providing such beautiful technique illustrations, and to those who helped to photograph our work. To all of the library staff and providers of literary resources, a big thank you for digging deep.

To our families, both human and animal, we thank you for providing us time away from home and play to complete this book. You have all helped to keep us focused on the goal of completion and were ever patient with the process. Lastly, we would like to thank the panel members of the 2011 AVMA Euthanasia Guidelines for laying the foundation for the improvement of euthanasia techniques as a whole.

Sincerely

Kathleen A. Cooney
Jolynn R. Chappell
Robert J. Callan
Bruce A. Connally

# Introduction

This book is written to be a practical guide for veterinarians, veterinary students, and technicians performing or assisting euthanasia, especially for the times they find themselves in unfamiliar situations. Hundreds of articles have been written on euthanasia over the century, but none of it has been collected in technical detail until now. When the first American Veterinary Medical Association (AVMA) Euthanasia Panel reported in 1963, the panel members drew from only 14 reference articles. By 2001's panel report, the number of published articles, presentations, and books utilized had grown to 223. The latest 2012 Euthanasia Panel Report took over 2 years to complete, utilizing the expertise of more than 70 individuals. All of this work, including that undertaken by the authors here, is done to ultimately prevent animal suffering, part of the veterinarian's oath, and when appropriate, offer support to the family/owner.

As with any movement forward in medicine, changes take time. Euthanasia is a very old term, Greek in origin, meaning "good death." The opposite is dysthanasia or "bad death." Understandably, these terms are quite subjective. The use of the term euthanasia can reflect the veterinarian's desire to do what is best for the animal and serves to bring about the best possible outcome for the animal (AVMA euthanasia guidelines draft review 2011). Another use is as a matter of humane technique only and not directly tied to the reason behind it, such as the euthanasia of laboratory animals.

Human caring for animals dates back to our earliest symbiotic partnering. For most of us, respect for life is instinctually understood and over the centuries, we have come to appreciate the anatomy and science of animals so much more. Pain mechanisms, animal behavior, and disease processes have been studied extensively, helping us to appreciate the level at which an animal might suffer. Philosophically speaking, we have come to some understanding of what an animal wants from life, its quality of life, and how it might view death itself.

The public's perception of euthanasia is very important, and careful consideration must be given to the manner of death in every circumstance. It must be addressed that the species being euthanized and the reasons for doing so can be vastly different. If the animal in question is being euthanized because of a terminal illness and suffering is imminent, the reason behind it is clear to most of us. When the animal in question is being euthanized for the use of its body, the reason why can become more difficult to understand, especially by those who oppose the killing of animals for production use. Whatever the reason for euthanasia, the procedure should be approached with respect to the animal and everyone involved.

In today's world, thanks in large part to the medical professionals who conducted studies over the last 100 years, we know ways to achieve as painless and anxiety-free a death as possible. With dedication to this line of work, these authors are certain that new techniques will emerge to make the euthanasia of animals even smoother, harboring fewer complications, and ultimately minimizing animal suffering and the ever-present concern of compassion fatigue.

If life is to be taken, it should be done with the utmost respect for the animal. Euthanasia is performed for a variety of reasons: an incurable disease, the conclusion of a terminal study, depopulation, and so on. Our responsibility is to make sure that the life is taken carefully and with great skill. For this reason, euthanasia must be performed by a veterinarian or, within the world of shelter and laboratory medicine, specially trained euthanasia technicians. We, the authors, hope this book increases knowledge of euthanasia to a whole new level. The chapters hold information on client considerations, sedation protocols, euthanasia techniques, aftercare options, and more. Each chapter includes species-specific teachings for easier reading and referencing. The euthanasia techniques themselves are divided into the various methods: inhalants, noninhalant pharmaceutical agents, and physical methods. This layout is similar to the AVMA's euthanasia guidelines for the expressed purpose of being easy to follow.

The methods listed within cause death by three basic mechanisms:

(1) Direct neuronal depression, that is, inhalant or noninhalant pharmaceutical agents.
(2) Hypoxia or displacing or removing oxygen, that is, inhaled gases, exsanguination.
(3) Physical disruption of brain activity, that is, decapitation, gunshot.

What method is chosen depends on the criteria listed below. The euthanasia techniques included in this book are evaluated using the following criteria (taken from the 2011 AVMA euthanasia guideline review):

- Ability to induce loss of consciousness and death without pain or anxiety.
- Time required to induce loss of consciousness.
- Reliability.
- Safety of personnel.
- Irreversibility.
- Compatibility with requirement and purpose.
- Documented emotional effect on observers and operators.
- Compatibility with use of tissue, examination.
- Drug availability and human abuse potential.
- Compatibility with species and health status.
- Ability to maintain equipment in working order.

- Safety for predators/scavengers should the body be consumed.
- Legal requirements.
- Environmental impacts of the method or carcass disposition.

Most euthanasia technique publications around the world use these criteria as their basis for acceptable methods. If a particular technique does not meet one or more criteria, the technique becomes conditionally acceptable, therefore negating some additional precaution to be taken. For example, an intracardiac injection of a barbiturate must be preceded by the administration of an anesthetic, because by itself, it will induce pain to the animal. Another example is the gunshot technique of a client-owned horse. This may have a great emotional effect for the observers, but when the safety of predators scavenging the body is considered, it may be necessary to do. The responsibility of the attending veterinarian is to examine all of these criteria and make the best judgment on how to proceed.

Because this book is meant to train veterinarians on euthanasia in the field and private practice, the authors have limited the range of techniques to those used routinely. The species covered include: dogs, cats, birds, pocket pets, common household reptiles and amphibians, horses, and livestock such as cattle, small ruminants, swine, and camelids. Therefore, we will not go into detail on euthanasia techniques used in laboratory medicine, wildlife control, and mass depopulation situations. For example, the use of inhalants is much broader within shelter and laboratory medicine and is, therefore, mentioned within on a much more focused level. Wonderful material has already been written on these topics and should be referenced accordingly. We also felt it beyond the scope of this book to discuss the human–animal bond in great detail. Anyone reading this book will undoubtedly understand the reasoning behind why we choose the techniques we do given the circumstances. When clients/owners are present, our goal is to support them, offering empathy and compassion at all times. For those of you performing the procedures, we acknowledge that compassion fatigue is very real and should not be ignored. Again, wonderful books have been written on these subjects and we recommend you explore the teachings within.

We hope you find this cohesive body of work highly informative and eye opening. These techniques are tried and true, used by us, the authors, and countless other colleagues who have shared their experiences. After reading, you should be able to perform these techniques with confidence. As with any type of medicine, practice solidifies your skills and we encourage you to continue learning as much about euthanasia as possible. Before performing euthanasia, veterinarians are required to learn the pharmacology, various techniques, and pet loss support required to ensure a stress- and pain-free passing for the pet and its family. The level of education in euthanasia depends a lot on the school attended, personal background, and continuing education. Technique manuals like this, bereavement training books, animal husbandry books, and drug formularies should be kept on file for quick referencing. It is important for veterinarians to recognize that advances are being made to improve the euthanasia experience from start to finish. New euthanasia drugs are being developed, new safer and faster techniques are being applied, and pet loss support is broadening.

Over the next 10 years, veterinary schools will undoubtedly be incorporating euthanasia technique training to better prepare new graduates entering the work force (Cohen-Salter and Folmer-Brown 2004). Families, production managers, and the public at large expect veterinarians to be trained in all euthanasia methods. May we exceed their expectations to the fullest.

# Chapter 1
# Client Considerations

Making the decision to end an animal's life can be extremely difficult for a client. Understanding the full scope of the reasons behind euthanasia before passing judgment as to whether it is ethically right or wrong is very important. Veterinarians can help clients determine if euthanasia is the best option for everyone. Veterinary training should provide the necessary tools to assess the animal and determine what physical changes the animal will endure as the end of life approaches. Age, disease, species, financial reserves, beliefs, etc., can all play a role in the decision to euthanize. The client may be considering euthanasia as the only possible option and it is the veterinarian's role to identify suffering and make sure all options are explored. Clients typically understand their animals very well, especially pertaining to quality of life, and their contributions to the conversation are crucial. The trick is not to let fear of the unknown be the guiding factor, but rather have logical reasoning and education as the prevailing rational.

The best way to approach end-of-life care is to set up the type of relationship with a client that has the best interests of the animal in view as the goal of treatment (Rollin 2006). This can be done early on in the veterinarian's communication with the family, long before a terminal diagnosis or any other reason for euthanasia presents. The client must feel safe talking to the veterinary staff regarding their fears, hopes, and plans for their animal's future. Professionalism and respect for the situation go a long way in demonstrating compassion. When death becomes imminent, except maybe in pure crisis situations, preparations and mutual understanding should already have been established. Suffering by the animal and client can hopefully be better avoided. With respect to this final decision, euthanasia is the treatment to end suffering (McMillan 2001).

Suffering is a very subjective term and difficult to define for any one situation. We must take all factors into consideration to help determine if suffering is occurring, and once recognized, how it can be lessened or stopped altogether through euthanasia. Many people look at suffering as the presence of constant pain that cannot be managed. Others view suffering as the inability to do what the heart desires. Both concepts are viable and can further be

*Veterinary Euthanasia Techniques: A Practical Guide*, First Edition. Kathleen A. Cooney, Jolynn R. Chappell, Robert J. Callan and Bruce A. Connally.
© 2012 John Wiley & Sons, Inc. Published 2012 by John Wiley & Sons, Inc.

classified as being physical and/or mental in nature. Suffering tends to remain a quality-of-life issue, regardless of the species.

Whether the animal in question is client owned or is kept for production-based purposes, the client will need to consider the following factors regarding disease before deciding to proceed forward with euthanasia:

- Is the animal free of pain?
- Can pain be controlled enough to make the animal comfortable and maintain a reasonable quality of life?
- Is the client willing to care for the animal in its current state of health?
- Is the animal maintaining good body weight and normal hydration?
- Is the client able/willing to finance procedures that would heal or at least improve the animal's condition?

Opening up dialog early in the end-of-life discussion is important so that everyone involved works together as a team and trust is established. Euthanasia is a viable option and should be addressed rather than skirting around the issue to avoid sadness by the caretakers. When euthanasia enters the discussion, the hope is that the client will feel safe talking about it and the veterinarian will understand their needs. In addition, it needs to be introduced delicately so that they do not feel that the veterinarian has given up prematurely (Cohen and Sawyer 1991). Ultimately, it is the disease or extenuating circumstance that is taking the pet's life. Veterinarians facilitate death when it is necessary and no other reasonable options are available. Once the decision to euthanize the animal has been made, it is time to talk to the client about the process. They may have very specific questions regarding the euthanasia that need to be addressed:

- What should I know about euthanasia?
- Can or should other animals be present?
- Where can euthanasia be done? (At the clinic, farm, in the home, etc.)
- Is euthanasia painful?
- Do I have to be present?
- How do we handle the body afterward?

The method of euthanasia should be discussed with the client before it is attempted. Many people understand the varying techniques that may be performed to achieve death, but just as many will not. Veterinarians can describe the technique of choice given the circumstances and still allow the client to voice any concerns they may have. It is important to reassure those present that the goal of euthanasia is to provide a stress-free and painless death. Explaining each step of the procedure will help ensure that there are no surprises that may be upsetting to the client. Some clients will choose not to be present during euthanasia, so details will have to be discussed beforehand.

Honesty as well as thoroughness is the key when talking about euthanasia so that unexpected situations are minimized. Financial concerns, quality of life, and matters of personal importance should be considered.

## Companion animals

An animal may be kept for companionship and a person's enjoyment, as opposed to livestock or working animals that are kept for economic or productive reasons. Pets, as they are commonly referred to, are euthanized everyday by the thousands in North America, including species such as dogs, cats, exotics, horses, and so on. Euthanasia is chosen for many reasons, such as debilitating age-related changes, life-limiting disease, financial limitations, safety risks, behavior issues, and so on. In practice, we hope to avoid "convenience euthanasia" as much as possible, and maintain this ultimate act of kindness for the sick and suffering.

Morally, veterinarians must examine all possible options before euthanasia is chosen. On a personal level, are we as members of the veterinarian field comfortable with the decision? Was the decision-making process thorough and were we motivated by proper reasoning? Professionally, did we offer every viable treatment or re-homing option? Are we acting in accordance with the law and feel certain that public opinion would show favorably on the decision to euthanize? Overall, veterinarians and attending staff may harbor guilt and resentment towards their decisions if the answers to these questions have not been well thought out. One may need to ask themselves if their reason for, and method of, euthanasia became public, would they feel certain events played out in the best interest of the animal and family.

Because of client/family dynamics, current medical options, public opinion, ethics, etc, veterinarians are encouraged to reach outside themselves for answers to difficult questions surrounding euthanasia. When appropriate, entire families can be consulted and viewpoints heard before euthanasia is chosen. Staff members can be brought into conversations so that life-maintaining options are not overlooked. Hasty decision-making can fuel compassion fatigue and 'burnout', leaving veterinary staff feeling troubled and upset.

When veterinarians and caregivers examine best and worst case scenarios, the goal is to arrive at euthanasia when it is most appropriate and justified. Someone just given a life-limiting diagnosis for their pet may view euthanasia as the worst-case scenario. They choose palliative and hospice care to provide more quality time; to allow the pet to remain with the hospice-devoted caretaker for as long as possible in the face of life-limiting disease. When managed appropriately, their goal might be a peaceful natural death at home. Euthanasia will be chosen when suffering is recognized regardless of strong palliative care, i.e. pain management, oxygen support, etc. While still recognizing its benefits, this family will view euthanasia as the worst-case scenario and endeavor away from it through hospice care as long as possible. Examining euthanasia as the best-case scenario, we might consider someone whose pet is diagnosed with a rapidly progressive incurable disease that is impossible to manage for numerous reasons. They do not have the time, physical ability, or financial resources to support a dying pet. Choosing euthanasia as the best-case scenario ultimately prevents suffering by all involved and allows them to be together to provide love and support for their pet during death. Therefore, they will endeavor towards euthanasia by acting on it sooner rather than later. To fully understand anyone's reasoning behind the decisions they make, veterinarians and support staff should appreciate all philosophical and logistical factors that may be present. It is also very important to recognize that the emotional implications of their decisions may remain with them forever, especially when guilt is involved.

In terms of a pet's disease, it is important to consider the pet's suffering as well as the client's. Can human caretakers safely move a large dog inside and outside for potty breaks? Are they emotionally strong enough to watch their horse worsen from lymphoma when it is the same cancer a human loved one died from? Can they financially handle the extreme cost of treatment for one cow and still provide for the rest of the herd and their client?

Also to consider is how much does the client understand about euthanasia. When euthanasia enters the conversation, the client may have a completely different scenario in mind than what will be done. Veterinarians or support staff can describe the procedure and address concerns of the client. If pain for the pet is the biggest concern, the client may be comforted to know that a sedative will be given first. If they are envisioning a gas chamber or something similar, they might be comforted to learn that it will be an injection, and so on. When euthanasia takes place in a shelter setting, and the client cannot be present, they might want to know standard protocol.

Educating clients about their options and how best to proceed is important so that, if they choose euthanasia for a beloved pet, they know that they are doing so for the right reasons. This will ultimately lessen the guilt and help them achieve healthier mourning (Wolfelt 2004).

Common questions by a client include the following:

- How do I know my pet is suffering?
- What does suffering look like?
- Does he have a good quality of life?
- Is it what my pet really wants?
- Is euthanasia the only option?
- What should I know about euthanasia?
- Is it important to have my kids present? Other pets?
- Where can euthanasia be done? In the clinic, home, or special center?
- Is euthanasia painful?
- Do I have to be present?
- How do I handle the body afterward?
- Will I be able to have a ceremony?
- How will I ever get over this loss?

The answers to these questions depend on many variables: beliefs, prior experiences (of the client and tending veterinarian), education, physical and mental fortitude, community offerings, etc. With regard to suffering, a quality-of-life assessment may be performed to help the client understand the changes that they are seeing in their pet. Factors such as hygiene, mobility, mentation, appetite, etc., are considered collectively to help a client determine how comfortable a dog or cat is in its body and surroundings (Villalobos and Kaplan 2007). If children will be present, they should be gently instructed on how euthanasia will occur and why. Children do remarkably well when introduced to euthanasia in a positive and safe manner (Cooney 2011). The presence of other pets may also be allowed if the client and veterinarian deem it appropriate. The location of the procedure depends on how the practice is designed and by what means veterinarians can accommodate a client's request. If the service can be performed in or near the client's home, they should be informed of that ahead of time. A memorial garden or comfort room may be perfect too.

A big concern for some clients is whether or not to be present when saying goodbye to a beloved pet. Many individuals find the act of euthanasia too emotional and thus feel they cannot be there. Like many of these questions, the answer is up to them. However, if they are leaving because they have a negative perception of the euthanasia procedure, veterinarians and staff can help them to understand exactly what will take place. Taking away the unknown can make the last moments with their pet more memorable and maintain the human-animal bond at its most critical time.

Once the decision has been made to proceed with euthanasia, there are numerous questions that need to be addressed by the tending veterinarian:

- What does the client need to know about euthanasia?
- Where should it take place?
- Who should be present?
- Has the body aftercare been decided?
- Is the person making the decision authorized to do so?
- Should a necropsy be chosen?
- Do we have any financial concerns or beliefs that need to be discussed?

Preparations for euthanasia will be made before the appointment and continue throughout to make sure that things proceed smoothly. The goal of those assisting with the procedure should be to make decisions on behalf of the client that will make their experience less stressful. It is comforting for them to know that the veterinary staff is working together to handle all arrangements.

Before gathering with the client and pet, everything should be ready to proceed. In the clinic setting, all drugs and equipment should be readied, the lights should be set to a comfortable level, and the staff alerted to the time and location of the euthanasia. There are usually many people involved with euthanasia in the hospital setting: receptionist, technician, doctor, and vet students where teaching is performed (Martin and Ruby 2004). In the field, those gathered may simply be the veterinarian and client, as is often the case on house calls. All drugs and supplies should be drawn, drugs recorded, and readied for the pet. If the setting and situation calls for personal touches such as candles, music, etc., everything should be in place. Clients may want to lay on the ground with smaller animals, so providing blankets, etc., can be a welcomed touch. It is important that everyone working in the area is alerted to the procedure, by verbal communication, a marker outside the door or area, etc. When possible, the surrounding area should be kept quiet to prevent distractions.

To allow the client more privacy, appointments can be scheduled during quieter times of the day, and handling payment and having forms signed beforehand can be helpful. More and more practices are gathering information and accepting payment over the phone, so it does not need to be discussed during the appointment. If practice policy is to have aftercare arrangements made ahead of time, such as a time for the crematory to pick up the pet afterward, this can all be done before euthanasia. It is important to be flexible, understanding, and compassionate to the client's wishes and emotions.

If the client chooses euthanasia outside of the clinic, for example, at their home, unique preparations need to be made. The attending veterinarian must carry all supplies with them to the pet being helped. Being prepared for every situation will help ensure a smooth procedure. Mobile veterinarians should have a good navigation system in place to ensure they arrive at the home on time. It is also helpful for clients to prepare themselves when you arrive by turning off phones and limiting distractions (Cooney 2011).

Following euthanasia, clients feel a wide range of emotions: sadness, anger, relief, guilt, helplessness, and more. Even if they have experienced the loss of a pet before, each time is unique and reflects directly upon the relationship they had with their animal. Veterinarians and their staff should know how to accurately discuss grief, offer guidance, and be informed on what the community can offer with aftercare options and pet loss support.

## Species-specific considerations

### Dogs and cats

According to the American Society for the Prevention and Cruelty to Animals (ASPCA), there were an estimated 75 million dogs and 85 million cats living in homes across the United States in 2011. A large percentage of people consider these animals to be the members of their family. Many are treated like surrogate children, and the pending loss of life can be overwhelming for those who have devoted so much love and time toward their care. With dogs and cats living close to home, usually in the home or within the confines of the property, the connection these two species have with their "people" could be considered unparallel to other species in today's society (Figure 1.1). Dogs and cats present unique challenges with regard to euthanasia, not because of any

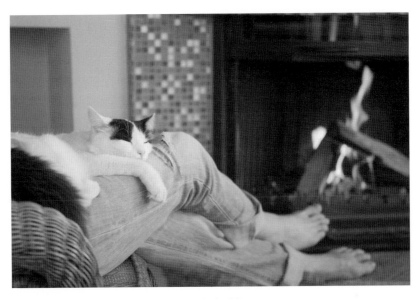

**Figure 1.1** A feline enjoying the comfort of its owner.

great anatomical differences, but rather because of the kinds of requests and wants that come from their human caretakers.

Because dogs and cats are so commonly intertwined with our daily life, clients commonly request unique locations for euthanasia. In the typical clinic setting, comfort rooms may be an option. In the home setting, requests such as "on the master bed" or "under the favorite tree in the backyard" are common. More elaborate requests may include "next to the lake frequented during hikes" or "in the motor-home the pet liked to travel in." Any place may be accommodated within reason as long as the euthanasia can be conducted safely and state regulations allow it.

Our pets develop lasting human relationships within the family and beyond, so it is common for friends and extended family to be present. For dogs and cats, this may include pet sitters, groomers, breeders, kennel attendants, and other veterinarians or vet technicians involved in the pet's care. For those people who may have a particularly difficult time with the loss, pet loss support personnel may also be present.

Many American households have more than one pet. This means that the client will need to decide if other pets are to be allowed to remain during the euthanasia procedure. The decision to allow another pet to remain in the area will depend on client beliefs, the temperament of both animals, the veterinarian's recommendations, etc. Ultimately, this is up to the client, unless other pets are disruptive to the procedure, wherein the veterinarian may suggest that the others be allowed in after the procedure to view the body.

How the euthanasia procedure itself is conducted can also be affected by dog and cat clients, commonly called pet parents. They may request pre-euthanasia sedation or anesthesia for their anxious dog or request an intraperitoneal injection for their cat because they want time to sit with them while they gently "slip away." Small animals can be euthanized on the client's lap, in their arms, etc., keeping the human–animal bond strong up until the end. These are matters that can be talked about before euthanasia is attempted. Actual euthanasia techniques will be described in Chapter 5.

Before death occurs, clients will need to know the common physical changes their dog or cat's body will undergo. They should be prepared for urination and defecation, possible agonal breathing, muscle fasciculation, etc., all of which will be discussed later. If they know what to expect, any changes they see will generally be acceptable, especially when they know that the actions are completely involuntary.

Whenever possible, aftercare arrangements, such as cremation or burial, should be determined before euthanasia. Dogs and cats can be easily trans-ported to a cremation facility of pet cemetery for internment or even buried on the client's property if local law permits. Large dogs can be moved using stretchers and smaller dogs and cats can be carried in blankets, towels, burial boxes, etc. As mentioned previously, dogs and cats commonly fill the role of surrogate children and clients may expect their bodies to be treated with the same level of respect as a human loved one. Veterinarians should strive to meet the level of care expected by the client.

## Exotics

Working with exotic companion animals has many rewards as well as many challenges. Their families often view these animals in different ways. They can be pets that are part of the family (Figure 1.2), or a less valued commodity that the client may not be willing to spend much money on for health care. Many clients want to help the animal within reasonable financial constraints and want to be sure the animal is not suffering. So many times, veterinarians are faced with the option of euthanasia simply due to the client's finances, even more so than with dogs and cats, especially when dealing with the small pocket pets such as hamsters, gerbils, and mice. These have a relatively short lifespan. Clients with fish of any species often value them as companion animals and share a human–animal bond similar to that seen between clients and other pets, such as dogs and cats (AVMA euthanasia guidelines draft review 2011). Actual euthanasia techniques will be described in Chapter 5.

Reptiles can survive a very poor state of health for extraordinarily long periods of time, so when they do arrive at the hospital, sometimes the only option is euthanasia. When medical care is a viable option, sometimes the amount of care they need or the home care required from the client is too much for the clients to take on and they decide on euthanasia.

Euthanizing almost any of the avian species is a very emotional ordeal in private practice. Birds are usually beloved pets and possibly have been part of the family for years, if not decades. This includes ducks and chickens, as these birds can become very special pets. The decision to euthanize can be very difficult and emotional, and veterinarians need to be there for our clients

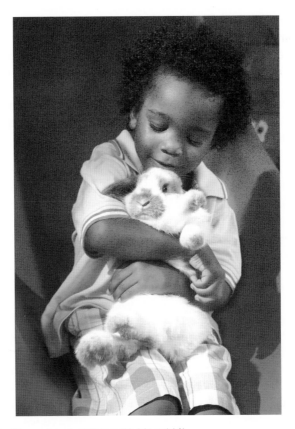

**Figure 1.2** Young boy bonding with his rabbit.

as guides to help them with their decision. The same guidelines as with other species should be followed such as quality of life, degree of pain or discomfort present, the ability of the client to care for the bird in its particular condition, and sometimes client financial concerns. Regardless of the reason, once the decision is made to end the life of the bird, the decision of whether the clients want to be present during the procedure and what form of body care is desired should all be made prior to the procedure. The clinician should offer a footprint or any feathers or leg band from the bird as a memorial of their pet. If the clients wish to be present during the euthanasia procedure, the steps involved should be explained prior to the procedure.

Another challenge is handling exotics and minimizing their stress in front of clients for the euthanasia procedure. Unfortunately, many exotic companion animals die before the client gets them into the hospital, either on the trip in or just after they have made the appointment. When this happens, the client may come to the conclusion that the trip into the veterinary hospital was just too stressful and that is what killed the pet. In reality, many people notice that their exotic pet is in need of medical care after it has been sick for quite some time. This can be due to the ability of the exotic pet to hide their symptoms for quite a long time, as a mode for survival. Other times, the client either is not aware that there is veterinary care available for these types of pets or they are unwilling to spend money on them and then decide too late that they better get them in for treatment. This commonly happens when the client has left the pet care in the hands of a child too young to make the decision on the pet's state of health. Whichever the case may be, birds and the small mammals such as hamsters and guinea pigs die before or just after their arrival to the hospital. If the ability of the exotic pet to reach the hospital setting for euthanasia is in question, then home visits may be more appropriate.

For those clients that do reach the clinic for euthanasia, minimizing stress is of the utmost importance. Whenever possible, exotics should be kept in familiar surroundings, such as a home cage and an aquarium. If the euthanasia procedure can be accomplished without removing them, this would be ideal for everyone. If physical contact is necessary, especially with regard to exotics that have had little human contact, a quiet environment setting and a rapidly performed euthanasia must be achieved.

There are varying thoughts on allowing other exotics to be present for the death of a companion. Opinions differ mostly because of the types of relationships that some exotics maintain and the length of time they have been together. With respect to birds, for example, a client may request that another bird be present during euthanasia. Birds are very sensitive and intelligent and can get quite stressed watching their companion die. When this is the concern, it may be prudent to recommend that the living bird view the body after euthanasia, but not be there for the actual process of euthanasia. Ultimately, the family will know what may be best for the remaining housemate. Another exotic pet, the rabbit, is also considered to be closely bonded to housemates. Clients may request that another rabbit be present or be allowed to spend time with the body afterward. Families have been known to borrow the body of the rabbit just euthanized to take home to the cage mate and then bring it back to the clinic the next day for aftercare such as cremation. Some members in the House Rabbit Society think that it helps the bonded mate get over the loss of their companion, so they recommend it.

It is not uncommon for some exotics to vocalize during a euthanasia proce-dure. This can alarm both the client and the clinician because they can happen suddenly and sometimes quite loudly. Two examples of this come from a stressed rabbit and hedgehog, both of which are generally very quiet animals with minimal vocalizations during life. If stressed during the euthanasia proce-dure, the hedgehog can make a sound similar to a young child screaming and the rabbit may give a piercing cry out. Generally though, if they are handled quietly and calmly, they will not get stressed. It is helpful to warn the client of this possible occurrence ahead of time. Again, pre-euthanasia sedation may help to lessen stress and subsequent vocalization.

Also, as with other types of companion animals, the exotic pet can continue with body movements long after the heart has stopped. In most of the species, the eyes do remain open and they do empty their bladders and bowels, so preparations for this may be made ahead of time. With birds, the eyes may close and the crop fluid will flow out of the mouth, especially if it was full prior to euthanizing. The veterinarian should always warn the client of all expected physical changes and verify when death has occurred.

## Horses

The position of the horse in society has evolved over the last half century from a working animal of primarily economic importance to a companion animal/pet whose economic value may be eclipsed by its personal value. It is essential that we know what relationship the client has with a horse before any other discussions take place. Veterinarians are commonly called to cattle ranches to euthanize a working animal and find tears in a tough old rancher's eyes when the horse has died.

There are many reasons to euthanize a horse (AAEP 2007). Trauma is a common reason and often requires an immediate decision for humane reasons. Advanced age, severe illness or lameness, and even economic conditions may be valid reasons for euthanasia. For some younger horse clients, this may be the first time they have had personal experience with death. For others, this horse may have been considered part of the family and may have been with the client for decades. If it is an emergency situation, the client, and possibly others in the vicinity, often have to make a decision quickly. Veterinary advice in these situations may be invaluable for the client to choose the most humane treatment for their animal (Lenz 2004). Actual euthanasia techniques will be discussed in Chapter 5.

The client may be considering euthanasia as only one possible option, when really several options may exist. One consideration is selling the animal for slaughter, which may ameliorate the financial loss incurred when a working animal is taken out of service. Currently, the value of a horse for slaughter is very low, due in part to legislation in 2007, which has forced closure of all equine slaughter plants in the United States (Heleski 2008). Horses sold for slaughter in the United States are transported to Canada or Mexico in the present system. This is not optimum for two reasons. First, the horses must be transported for long distances to reach a slaughter facility. Second, and perhaps more important, veterinarians have no control over slaughter procedures utilized in these plants (Cordes 2008). As this book is being written, several states are pursuing legislation that would legalize horse slaughter. The result of this legislative effort is hard to predict in the current political climate. If slaughter is legalized again in the United States, it would increase the base value of horses and give clients a viable means of recovering some of the investment they have made in their working animal (Heleski 2008). An active horse slaughter industry would also decrease the very real problem of equine carcass disposal in the United States.

Another consideration is the well-trained horse that has become physically unable to perform his work. This horse might be sold to another person who requires a much lower level of performance. It is also possible to find organizations such as therapeutic riding groups who will be able to use a gentle, dependable horse that cannot otherwise perform as a higher level athlete.

Donations to these groups may have significant tax advantages for the horse client as well. Of overwhelming concern in these situations is the horse's comfort. A seriously injured horse may not be able to be used humanely, even at the lowest levels of performance.

Clients may choose to breed a very valuable animal, which has been injured, before considering euthanasia. Their motives may be to either recoup some of their loss or to perpetuate a loved companion. These situations need to be looked at carefully to ascertain if this is a humane use of this animal or if immediate euthanasia is a better option for the horse. New enhanced reproductive techniques may now allow harvesting of eggs or sperm immediately after euthanasia in certain situations.

Once the decision is made, it is time to talk to the client about the process. The client may have a very strong preference for the method of euthanasia used, and the veterinarian will need to work to accommodate their wishes within the bounds of humane euthanasia. For example, some owners may request a physical method of euthanasia rather than an injection so the horse may be allowed to biodegrade naturally; give the body back to nature if you will without risking secondary wildlife death from barbiturate ingestion. They will need to know why a captive bolt gun is being used or why it is important to euthanize close to an area with vehicle access. Moving a deceased horse has many challenges that must be considered before death occurs. More on equine aftercare specifics will be discussed in Chapter 6.

Some clients may ask if euthanasia will be painful for the horse or if the horse will be stressed or afraid. Veterinarians can reassure them that the goal is to make the procedure as quiet and painless as possible for the horse and for the client. Each step of the procedure can be discussed so there are no surprises that may be upsetting to the client and those present.

Some clients will choose to be absent when the euthanasia is performed. This is a legitimate choice, which may actually make the process easier for the veterinarian and the horse. A very emotional client can transfer their anxiety to the horse. If they do choose to observe the euthanasia, it is important to talk about what they will see.

Almost all horses will be standing when euthanized. They will generally not just lie down and shut their eyes, but will lose consciousness and fall to the ground. This abrupt crash to the ground can be the most troubling part of equine euthanasia. In some hospital situations, an anesthesia induction stall may be used to mitigate the fall. This appears more acceptable to the horse client but may not be better for the horse. Many horses will become anxious in this very confining space. It is important for the client to understand that when the horse falls it is unconscious and, therefore, will not feel anything or be afraid. Even though the horse will be unconscious, the heart will continue to beat for several minutes. The veterinarian must stay and monitor the horse until all signs of life are gone.

Human bodies are always presented with eyes closed at funerals. Many horse clients are startled and troubled when the horse dies with eyes wide open. Veterinarians often forget that open eyes are equated with

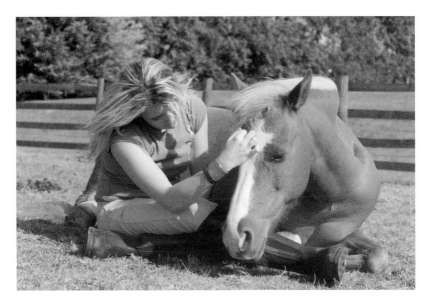

**Figure 1.3** Woman and her horse. This close proximity during euthanasia is not safe and should be avoided. Time for bonding should be allowed before the procedure begins.

consciousness, and perhaps even fear, by some horse clients. It is important to take the time to explain this to the client and reassure them the horse is not aware.

Because it is unnatural for a horse to fall down, this may startle other horses in the area. Some clients want the other horses to understand that their herd mate is gone. Some horses will actually try to get the euthanized horse up by nuzzling or pawing at it. Other horses will completely ignore the deceased horse. Most horses come investigate for a short time and then go on as if nothing can be done. Whatever the expected reaction, horses can be allowed to watch as long as they can do so safely.

## Companion Livestock

Some commercial livestock have value to the client that goes beyond simple commercial dollar value. This may be true for special seed stock animals, show or 4H animals, or pet livestock. In these cases, treatment and euthanasia decisions can become very complex. Appreciating the emotional ties a client may have with the animal become very important in the communication process (Figure 1.4). Clients may request treatment and care that is beyond the ordinary. There are also clients of pet livestock that do not feel comfortable with euthanasia of their pet and will request supportive care that provides as much comfort to the animal as possible until it passes away naturally. These requests often challenge the livestock veterinarian and, in some cases, test our beliefs in the client's ability to minimize animal suffering and provide animal welfare, including a humane death.

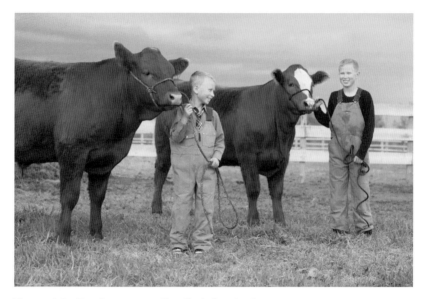

**Figure 1.4** Two boys presenting their livestock.

## Production animals

An important aspect of livestock production and veterinary medicine is rec-ognizing animal suffering and providing a humane end of life for animals that have serious or terminal disease. Livestock including cattle, sheep, goats, pigs, llamas, alpacas, and more all fall into this category. This section will focus on the specific considerations and methods of euthanasia for livestock species and is meant to augment the information provided in the American Veterinary Medical Association (AVMA) Guidelines on Euthanasia.

There are many factors that go into the decision of whether an animal should be euthanized. In the livestock production setting, this will include the type and severity of disease, the likelihood of recovery from disease, the degree of recovery expected and the potential for persistent complications and suffering, and the prognosis for return to function or productivity. In addition to the health and animal wellness issues, veterinarians and producers are also faced with the evaluation of the economics of treatment relative to the predicted return to production.

A simple but effective method of economic decision-making is to evaluate the replacement value of the animal relative to the prognosis for return to productivity and the cost of treatment. On strictly economic terms, further treatment of an animal is economically justified if:

[Replacement Value] × [Prognosis] > [Cost of Treatment]

For commercial livestock operations, it is evident that more complicated medical conditions generally have a lower prognosis and higher cost of treatment resulting in less incentive to treat the animal. In these cases, culling or, if necessary, euthanizing the animal should be considered. In some circumstances, the animal has already been treated with medications that have meat-withholding periods and the animal cannot be immediately salvaged for slaughter. Such cases may present difficult dilemmas regarding the cost of further treatment, prolonged drug withdrawal times, or continued suffering of the animal if treatment is withdrawn to allow for elimination of drug residues. In some cases, further treatment is not warranted and salvage for slaughter is not an option due to the animal being recumbent, having drug residues, or having a disease that would not be acceptable for slaughter. In such cases, the decision for euthanasia is often the most humane choice (Figure 1.5).

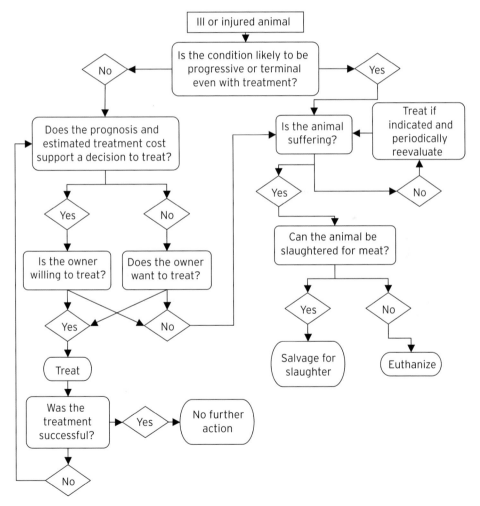

**Figure 1.5** Determining factors for the euthanization of livestock. (Robert Callan, author.)

Some indications for euthanasia include the following:

- Fractured leg, where treatment is not considered a suitable option.
- Severe trauma.
- Progressive or nonresponsive infectious disease (pneumonia, pleuritis, peritonitis, mastitis, metritis, enteritis, etc.).
- Inability to stand or walk.
- Zoonotic disease with significant public health implications (i.e., rabies).
- Unresponsive metabolic disease resulting in debilitation.
- Progressive organ failure (heart, liver, kidney).
- Persistent pain or discomfort (suffering) that is not responsive to medical treatment.

The question of whether or not an animal is suitable for market and slaughter is sometimes difficult. Beef quality assurance guidelines recommend that animals should not be marketed for meat unless they:

- do not pose a known public health threat;
- have cleared proper drug withdrawal times;
- do not have a condition that would result in condemnation at slaughter, such as severe infectious disease, advanced neoplasia, or unresponsive metabolic disease;
- are able to ambulate and are able to remain standing for transportation;
- are not severely emaciated (body condition score >2.5/9 for beef cattle or >1/5 for dairy cattle);
- do not have a uterine or vaginal prolapse with visible fetal membranes;
- do not have advanced stages of ocular neoplasia (eye cancer, ocular squamous cell carcinoma);
- do not have advanced lumpy jaw.

Most livestock producers are very familiar with terminal disease in their animals and the decisions leading up to euthanasia. As some producers put it, "If you own livestock, you quickly learn about dead stock." Livestock producers are routinely very knowledgeable about basic medical conditions in their animals, fundamental care, and treatment. In addition, most livestock producers generally demonstrate a strong sense of animal welfare and are conscientious at minimizing animal suffering in the face of illness or injury.

The initial consideration with the client is whether or not euthanasia is an appropriate decision. Once the decision for euthanasia is made, it is important to discuss the method of euthanasia and what the client should expect from the procedure. When working with a regular client, the method of euthanasia has often already been established. However, with new clients or clients that own pet livestock, this is a very important discussion. There are two basic options for euthanasia in livestock: euthanasia by lethal injection of a pentobarbital solution, or euthanasia by rendering the animal unconscious with penetrating impact (captive bolt or gunshot) to the head, followed, if necessary, by a secondary means to cause cardiac or respiratory arrest. Both methods have their advantages and disadvantages and must be discussed with the client when the method of euthanasia has not been previously established.

Euthanasia by injection of a pentobarbital solution often is considered a more aesthetically acceptable method of euthanasia than gunshot or captive bolt. However, the cost of the procedure may be considerably more due to the cost of the euthanasia drugs, particularly in larger livestock such as cattle. There may also be additional costs associated with the placement of an intravenous catheter if this is deemed necessary. If euthanasia by injection of pentobarbital is selected, then the carcass remains must be disposed of in a way that prevents scavenger animals (dogs, coyotes, wolves, bears, eagles, etc.) from consuming any of the tissues. This means that the carcass must be quickly picked up by the renderer, buried, or properly ensiled to prevent toxicity and possible death in scavenger animals.

Euthanasia by gunshot or captive bolt may have negative aesthetic connotations with some people, particularly pet livestock clients, or when used on neonates and young stock. While this may be difficult to explain in rational terms, it is still the perception of many clients and veterinarians. As will be discussed, proper euthanasia by gunshot or captive bolt renders the animal immediately unconscious with less physical or psychological effects caused by the prolonged restraint and time for venipuncture that is required for intravenous administration of pentobarbital solution.

It is always good to ensure that the client understands the fundamental goals of euthanasia. A well-performed euthanasia will rapidly render the animal unconscious in a humane way with minimal physical pain or psychological stress. This is followed by cardiac and respiratory arrest. For inexperienced clients, it may be useful to describe the procedure in detail prior to performing the euthanasia so that they know what to expect and may also be prepared for any adverse responses. For example, if euthanizing an animal by pentobarbital injection, the client should be informed that the animal will become unconscious rapidly after the injection and will become recumbent. There may be some persistent paddling of the legs. Respiratory arrest generally precedes cardiac arrest but this can take up to 5 minutes. During that time, the animal may demonstrate several deep breaths. In ruminants and camelids, the loss of esophageal tone following euthanasia will often result in spontaneous passive regurgitation following death. Spontaneous urination and defecation may also occur.

When gunshot or captive bolt is used, the animal is instantaneously rendered unconscious and will become immediately recumbent. This is more dramatic than with pentobarbital euthanasia, and the client should be forewarned, particularly if they are observing or assisting with the restraint of the animal. Unconsciousness can be demonstrated by the lack of a corneal reflex. Hemorrhage is often observed from the penetrating wound. Nasal hemorrhage (epistaxis) may also be observed. While the animal is rendered immediately unconscious, cardiac or respiratory arrest may not occur right away and secondary methods (pithing, exsanguination, intravenous potassium chloride, and pneumothorax) are often used to ensure rapid death. During this time, the animal may show persistent paddling that can increase with time until final death. This is often more pronounced compared with euthanasia by pentobarbital because the penetrating concussion to the brain, while rendering the animal unconscious, does not prevent involuntary motor activity of the extremities. Further, the penetrating concussion disrupts the motor inhibitory centers of the brain making spontaneous peripheral motor responses and reflexes more exaggerated.

The physical location of the euthanasia may also be a consideration for the client and the veterinarian. Should euthanasia be performed on the farm or at a veterinary facility? If the animal is recumbent or would have difficulty being transported, a farm euthanasia may be preferred. The client may request an on-farm euthanasia for pure convenience. This must be balanced with the availability of suitable restraint for the animal in order to perform the procedure in a safe manner. Options for disposal of the carcass must also be considered. In the cases of acute skeletal trauma or fracture, the client may request on-site slaughter. Alternatively, the animal may be picked up by the renderer, buried or ensiled on site, or sent to a veterinary diagnostic laboratory for necropsy. If the client would like a necropsy, this can be performed on the farm following the euthanasia. If the client requests that a necropsy be performed at a veterinary diagnostic laboratory, it may be easier to load the animal onto a trailer alive and then transport to the diagnostic laboratory for evaluation, euthanasia, and necropsy.

# Chapter 2
# Equipment

**W**hen preparing to perform euthanasia, it is imperative that all the necessary equipment, drugs, and miscellaneous supplies are ready to help ensure that things proceed smoothly. Whether in the clinic or out in the field, having a variety of equipment close at hand will allow you to perform whichever euthanasia technique is most appropriate given the patient and setting. The types of drugs and supplies to keep will depend on the veterinarian's preferred method of euthanasia, the type of animal, the presence of onlookers, the location, etc. For example, most veterinarians choose to euthanize dogs and cats via an intravenous (IV) injection of a noninhalant pharmaceutical agent, and therefore, needles, catheters, and syringes are needed. Within the shelter setting, other techniques may be utilized, such as the inhalation of gas mixtures, and specialized equipment must be maintained to ensure the safety of animal and personnel (Rhoades 2002). Large chambers and other such equipment for this method are very specific to inhalant agents and will not be commonly found in veterinary clinics. Whatever the method, all supplies need to be on location and ready to use by those specifically trained to perform technically proficient euthanasia. The majority of explanation behind the use of all types of equipment can be found in Chapter 5.

For the more uncommon techniques used in private practice, such as immersion of amphibians in euthanasia solutions, the equipment needed will be described in the pertinent sections within this chapter.

## Technique-specific equipment

### Inhalant techniques

### Equipment List

| | |
|---|---|
| Facemask | Rope gauze or string |
| Gas chamber | Inhalant drugs |
| Flow meters | Cotton balls |
| Gas filtration system | |

*Veterinary Euthanasia Techniques: A Practical Guide*, First Edition. Kathleen A. Cooney, Jolynn R. Chappell, Robert J. Callan and Bruce A. Connally.

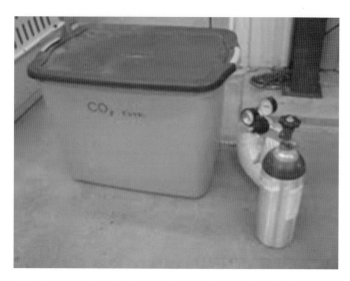

**Figure 2.1**  Example of a simple gas chamber for small animals.

The use of inhalant anesthetics and gases as the primary means of euthanasia are considered acceptable and conditionally acceptable for small dogs, cats, and some exotics. Their use may not be ideal when owners are present, especially when the animal must be placed in a chamber creating a forced physical separation between the pet and owner (Figure 2.1; American Veterinary Medical Association (AVMA euthanasia guidelines draft review 2011). If the pet can be safely held close to the owner while receiving an inhalant such as isoflurane, this should be allowed. Facemasks of various sizes should be kept to accommodate different head sizes. A preattached strap or added rope is needed to secure the mask over the animal's nose. Cotton balls soaked in anesthetic liquids may be placed within masks or chambers to facilitate inhalation by the animal.

Gas chambers must be of high quality and free of defects (Figure 2.2). Defects are a danger to personnel and will increase the time to achieve euthanasia. The inhalant gases should be properly filled before use and waste captured in a scavenging unit, keeping in mind that some gases should only be infused once the animal is already inside the chamber. They should allow for separation of animals if more than one will be euthanized at a time. They should be easy to clean and be free of odor whenever possible. The chamber must be in a ventilated area, preferably even outside where permitted, and well lit for animal observation. When indoors, hazardous gas monitors should be present and maintained to alert staff to possible gas leaks into the air. The use of flow meters will help ensure that gases are delivered at optimal rates and levels. If concentrations are not ideal for the inhalant, the animal may experience distress. Carbon monoxide (CO) is flammable, and therefore, any electrical equipment in the area must be spark free and explosion proof (AVMA euthanasia guidelines draft review 2011).

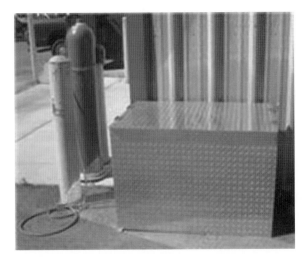

**Figure 2.2** Example of a simple gas chamber for small animals.

## Noninhalant pharmaceutical agent injections

### Equipment List

| | |
|---|---|
| Catheters | Syringes |
| Needles | Male adaptors |
| Extension sets | Tape |
| 4×4 gauze | Saline |
| Hydrogen peroxide | Tourniquet |
| Drugs | Sharps container |
| Clippers | |

These items are commonly used for the administration of injectable euthanasia agents. As of 2012, all noninhalant injectable agents must be given either directly in the vein, within the abdomen, or within organs that will rapidly move the drug toward the site of action. How these items are used depends on the veterinarian's method of choice and the animal being euthanized.

Depending on the species, IV administration can be accomplished using direct venipuncture with needles or by placing an IV catheter. When the injection is performed in the leg or arm of the animal, a tourniquet may be used to occlude blood flow and increase the size of the vein. Clippers may be used to remove hair from over the injection site improving visibility. Saline is often used to flush an IV catheter to ensure proper placement. Syringes may be luer-lock or non-luer-lock. When a highly viscous euthanasia solution is administered, the luer-locking tip is recommended to avoid leakage. IV extension sets and male adaptors may be used to stop the backflow of blood from catheters. Gauze and hydrogen peroxide can be used to clean the injection site before and after euthanasia. A sharps container is required for proper disposal of needles, catheter stylets, etc. The size of needles, syringes, and catheters is directly related to the size of the animal.

## Physical methods

### Gunshot

> **Equipment List**
>
> Appropriate firearm
> Cartridge of appropriate type for species
> Halter or other method of head restraint
> Ear and eye protection

Handguns, rifles, or shotguns can all be used for euthanasia of livestock, including horses. Handguns have the advantage of being compact and easy to store. Handguns are ideal for euthanasia at very close range (2-10 in.). Rifles and shotguns may also be used at close range or at much longer ranges in special circumstances. Rifles provide acceptable accuracy and effective euthanasia at longer distances, especially when fitted with a telescopic scope. The AVMA guide discourages euthanasia via gunshot to the chest, as death is not instantaneous. This method may still be utilized in wild animals where approach is impossible. A competent marksman can shoot an animal in the head at considerable distance but this requires much practice.

The caliber, type of bullet, and muzzle velocity all affect the suitability of a firearm for euthanasia. The competency of the operator is also important when euthanizing an animal with a firearm. Larger, more powerful firearms will cause more tissue damage and thus may allow for minor placement errors. Even a very large and powerful weapon will not compensate for poor bullet placement.

Some veterinarians have extensive experience euthanizing animals with firearms, but others will not and are encouraged to get advice from an experienced firearm professional before purchasing a gun for use in euthanasia. There are literally hundreds of choices of pistols, rifles, and shotguns on the market, which could be employed for euthanasia. Some will be better than others. Multiply this by the hundreds of bullet choices used in these weapons and the options become limitless. Training in firearm safety and use of the weapon is essential to prevent injury, accidents, and suffering.

Many mobile large animal veterinarians are reluctant to own or carry a firearm or captive bolt gun with them in their vehicle due to regulatory, theft, and safety concerns. Depending upon local regulations, the veterinarian may need to possess a concealed firearm permit to carry the weapon in the vehicle and may also be limited to only using a firearm for euthanasia outside of city limits. While the upfront cost for a firearm is less than a captive bolt gun, a firearm is associated with greater liability. Firearm safety training is highly recommended before using a firearm for euthanasia. In addition, there is a greater concern of theft with firearms versus captive bolt guns.

Choosing the appropriate caliber and bullet type is important for effective stunning and killing when using a firearm for euthanasia (Figure 2.3). Using a

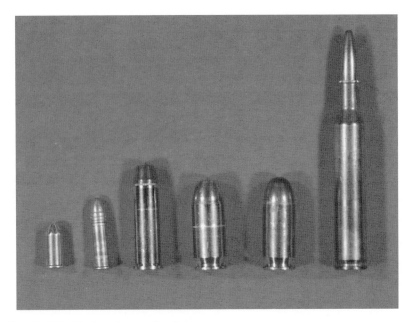

**Figure 2.3** Various types of bullets.

firearm caliber and bullet type that has a lower effective energy may result in rendering the animal unconscious, but may not effectively result in cardiac and respiratory arrest, and death. In such cases, secondary methods of causing cardiac and respiratory arrest such as pithing, exsanguination, IV potassium chloride (KCl), or pneumothorax (livestock) should be performed once the animal is unconscious.

Shotguns can also be used as effective firearms for euthanizing larger animals such as horses and livestock. When using a shotgun with birdshot, the damage from multiple projectiles is often more severe than that induced by a single bullet from a pistol or rifle. All firearms are loud and can cause hearing damage. The loudness is accentuated in enclosed spaces. There is also the risk of eye trauma from debris or fragments with all firearms. Ear and eye protection should always be worn when using firearms for euthanasia.

**Captive bolt**

### Equipment List

Captive bolt gun, bolt, and cartridge
*Secondary equipment*:
   Pithing instrument
   Sharp necropsy knife, at least 6 in. long
   Scalpel blade and handle
   Noninhalant injectable agents and supplies
   Halter or other method of head restraint

**Table 2.1** Recommended firearm and cartridge for euthanasia of livestock.

| Firearm | Animal type | Caliber | Bullet |
| --- | --- | --- | --- |
| Handgun or rifle | Calves, sheep, goats | .22 5.5 mm | Soft or hollow point |
| | Pigs <100 kg | .22 5.5 mm | Round nose |
| | Adult cattle (>24 months) | .22 magnum .357 9 mm | Round nose Soft or hollow point Soft or hollow point |
| | Horses | .357 9 mm | Soft or hollow point Soft or hollow point |
| | Adult bulls, pigs > 100 kg | .357 9 mm | Round nose Round nose |
| Shotgun | Calves, sheep, goats | 20, 16, or 12 gauge | #4, 5, or 6 birdshot |
| | Pigs <100 kg | 20, 16, or 12 gauge | #4, 5, or 6 birdshot |
| | Adult cattle | 16 or 12 gauge | Slug or #4 or 5 birdshot |
| | Horses | 16 or 12 gauge | Slug or #4 or 5 birdshot |
| | Adult bulls, pigs > 100 kg | 12 gauge | Slug or #4 or 5 birdshot |

*Source*: Adapted from Welfare aspects of animal stunning and killing methods (2004) *European Food Safety Authority* AHAW/04-027. Scientific report of the Scientific Panel for Animal Health and Welfare on a request from the commission related to welfare aspects of animal stunning and killing methods.

There are several equipment-related factors that must be considered by veterinarians choosing to use a firearm or captive bolt gun for euthanasia. A fundamental criterion for the humane euthanasia of animals by gunshot or captive bolt stunner is to render the animal immediately unconscious (<1 second) followed by cardiac and respiratory arrest. When the captive bolt does not accomplish euthanasia by itself, a secondary method must be applied.

The tip of the penetrating captive bolt is concave with a sharp edge that makes it easier for the bolt to penetrate the skull and enter the calvarium. The amount of concussive force and brain damage is in part determined by the mass, diameter, length, and velocity of the bolt upon firing. These characteristics vary between captive bolt stunners and thus determine their suitability for different size and species of animal (Table 2.1). The length of the bolt varies from 57 to 136 mm, with diameters from 12 to 14 mm. Bolt velocity is about 60 m/s (200 ft/s) with a kinetic energy of around 295 ft lb (400 J).

Both trigger-operated and contact-firing captive bolt stunners are available (Figure 2.4). Both pistol and cylindrical models are available. The trigger-operated captive bolt guns seem to allow for more control of placement over the target.

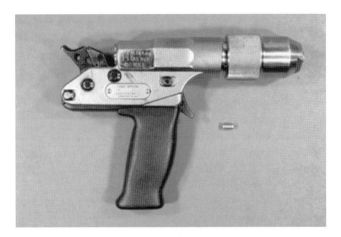

**Figure 2.4**  Example of a trigger-operated penetrating captive bolt stunner. This model is the Cash Special manufactured by Accles & Shelvoke.

For field use, captive bolt stunners are powered by a blank cartridge, generally .22 or .25 caliber. They require routine cleaning between use to ensure that the bolt moves freely and has adequate velocity. The bolt must be fully retracted into the barrel after each shot. The rubber buffer rings contained in the cylinder regulate the penetration depth and also retract the bolt out of the head after firing. These must be inspected and replaced periodically. The bolt should also be inspected regularly and replaced if it is bent or damaged (Figure 2.5).

Several trigger-operated penetrating captive bolt stunners are available in multiple models including the Cash Special, Blitz-Kerner, Magnum 25, and the Schermer stunners. Trigger-operated captive bolt stunners come in both pistol and cylindrical designs. The two different designs have different ergonomics such that the cylindrical design is easier to use in standard slaughter kill boxes

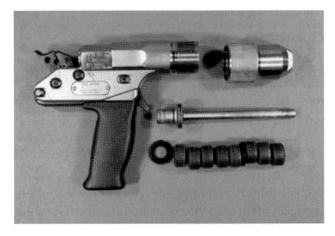

**Figure 2.5**  The Accles & Shelvoke Cash Special disassembled for cleaning and inspection of the penetrating bolt and the buffer rings.

from above the animal. In the field, cylindrical models can be comfortably used from the side of the animal, but are more awkward from directly in front of the animal. The pistol design is easiest to use from in front of the animal or to the side.

The greatest drawback of a captive bolt stunner is the initial monetary investment as the cost of these devices currently ranges from $350 to $3350 (2011 prices). However, shells for these stunners cost less than $0.20 each, and it is estimated that the cost over the life of the equipment is less than $1.00 per euthanasia with proper maintenance. Its greatest advantages over firearms are that captive bolt stunners are generally safer for the operator and bystanders, do not require special licensing, and can be used within city limits.

When properly used on various species, the captive bolt stunner will effectively render the animal immediately unconscious, but may not cause sufficient damage to critical areas of the brain to result in cardiac and respiratory arrest, and death. It is important that ancillary equipment be on site to complete euthanasia via a secondary method by inducing cardiac and respiratory arrest. Typical methods used in animals include pithing, exsanguination, IV or intracardiac injection of saturated KCl solution, or pneumothorax. The pithing rod can be any sturdy rod, preferably with a handle, at least 6 in. long. Many common instruments can be used as reusable pithing rods including a long screwdriver, Buhner needle, or even a long nail. Disposable pithing rods are also available (www.pithingrods.com). These are flexible plastic rods approximately 1 m in length.

Exsanguination requires a sturdy sharp knife, preferably with a blade at least 6 in. in length. Some practitioners will alternatively cut the abdominal aorta and vena cava via rectal palpation using a scalpel. Cardiac arrest, followed by respiratory arrest, can be achieved by injection of a lethal amount of KCl as well.

Terminal hypoxia can be achieved by inducing a pneumothorax in the unconscious animal, typically livestock. This is accomplished by performing a deep intercostal incision into the thorax over at least two-thirds of the intercostal space with a knife or scalpel blade.

## Decapitation

### Equipment List

Anesthetic agent
Cutting shears
Guillotine
Sharp knife
*Secondary equipment:*
  Pithing rod

Decapitation is a conditionally acceptable method of euthanasia in small rodents and birds when they are anesthetized and an adjunctive method in other species. Decapitation using a heavy shears or guillotine is effective for some species. Because the central nervous system of reptiles and amphibians is tolerant to hypoxic and hypotensive conditions (Cooper 1989), decapitation must be followed by pithing or another method of destroying brain tissue (Wright, KM. 2001). Decapitation should only be performed as part of a three-step euthanasia protocol (injectable or inhaled anesthetic, decapitation, and pithing).

## Cervical dislocation

### Equipment List

Anesthetic agent
Thin cylindrical/rod-shaped device

Cervical dislocation is a conditionally acceptable method of euthanasia by the AVMA for unconscious small mammals, birds, and reptiles, and is acceptable in turkeys. In this method, a small board, dowel, or pencil (depending on the size of animal) is placed at the base of the animal's skull. Exact description of this technique will be in Chapter 5.

## Rapid Freezing

### Equipment List

Anesthetic agent
Liquid nitrogen
Tongs

Reptiles, amphibians, companion arthropods, and baby mice can be euthanized by rapid freezing in liquid nitrogen, which results in immediate death. To be considered conditionally acceptable, species undergoing rapid freezing must be <4 kg (Close 1997) and be unconscious or presumed dead already. The AVMA views it as an adjunctive method. Most private practice facilities do not house liquid nitrogen, so this is not considered a common method of euthanasia for small animals; however, it is worth mentioning for those who do keep it on site; that is, reproduction laboratories, dermatology centers, etc.

## Miscellaneous

### Equipment List

| | |
|---|---|
| Bandage scissors | Hemostats |
| Rubber gloves | Towels/blankets |
| Stethoscope | Stretcher |
| Flashlight | Drug box and key |
| Trash container | Sharps container |
| Skin adhesive | Supply bag |
| Clay paw prints | Pet loss literature |
| Kleenex | Calculator |
| Body bags/boxes | Restraint devices |

These miscellaneous supplies aid in the euthanasia appointment itself (Figure 2.6). A stethoscope to auscult the heart and cardiac arrest is still considered the gold standard for confirming death even though other death indicators may be present. Some practices/shelters may use long needles and syringes for the cardiac-puncture test to check for cardiac standstill (Rhoades 2002). Rubber gloves can be worn to protect hands from bodily fluids and infectious diseases. Towels and blankets soften the area for small animals and, when tucked under the body, can catch urine and feces following death. They can also be used to help restrain fractious animals. Flashlights are important when visibility is poor. A calculator should be on hand to calculate drug doses. Liquid skin adhesives can be used to secure catheters to the skin in large animals and close the eyelids of the deceased.

Restraint equipment should always be carried in case the animal being euthanized requires more handling than expected. This equipment is meant to aid the administrator by keeping the animal in a stable position allowing for a safer euthanasia procedure. Such equipment could be muzzles, halters, cat bags, squeeze shoots, etc. Even sedation/anesthetic drugs can be considered restraint equipment. If the animal being euthanized cannot be adequately restrained, and the risk to animal or handler is too great, euthanasia may need to be postponed until circumstances are improved.

In the field setting, a supply bag is necessary to hold equipment along with a drug box and key. Following euthanasia, a stretcher may be needed to move a midsized animal and body bags or boxes used to transport the animal home for burial or to the crematory. A trash or sharps container is important to have so that medical waste is not left behind.

Family support is also important. Kleenex should be kept in the area for client-present euthanasia and pet loss literature offered. Pet loss keepsakes such as clay footprints are very popular and may soon be considered standard practice (Cooney 2011). Any item that the veterinarian and staff feels may be helpful to the client should be kept close and ready to use.

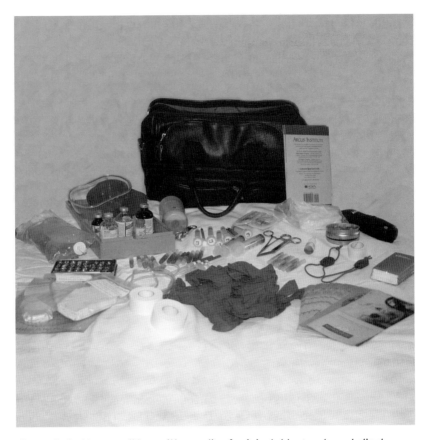

**Figure 2.6** House call bag with supplies for injectable agents and client support.

## Euthanasia area equipment

Reliability, repeatability, and safety are vital with euthanasia procedures. Personnel safety is imperative when working with euthanasia drugs, equipment, and sick, and potentially fractious animals. The euthanasia area should have good lighting for the veterinarian to accurately perform the desired technique. Euthanasia equipment and supplies should be housed in a safe place and kept free of defects. When wear and tear is becoming evident, such as a tourniquet that loses its tightening capabilities or a facemask that leaks, items like these should be replaced. In fact, two of every item should be kept in case its immediate use is needed.

An eye-wash station should be close by in the case of accidental eye contact with euthanasia drugs. Treatment areas are often very busy and crowded. Adequate space to work should be sought out and used needles and syringes should be properly disposed of in sharps containers.

When practical, a euthanasia room or area should be established to limit contact with other animals and people. Many small animal clinics today have

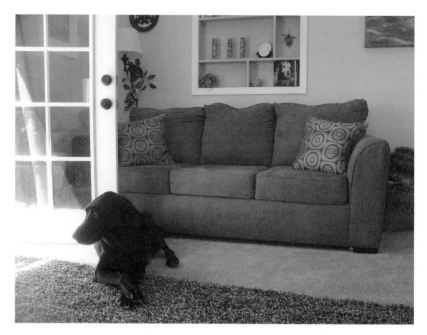

**Figure 2.7** Comfort room.

"comfort rooms" to allow clients to gather with their pets (Figure 2.7). While these rooms are designed to be pleasant for families, they should still provide the necessary equipment. Euthanasia procedure areas should contain a safe surface to work on, such as a floor or table. It should hold a first-aid kit, cleaning supplies, and animal-restraint devices such as muzzles, collars, and leashes, or feline-restraint bags tucked out of site and ready for use. Restraining devices are not ideal to use when the family is present, but having them close by eliminates stressful waiting while staff retrieves what they need from another room.

Due to the desired outcome of death, sterility for the patient is not a concern. There is a concern, however, for other living pets that may enter the area or be treated with the same equipment for other procedures. When euthanasia is conducted in a general clinic treatment area, all surfaces should be disinfected following the procedure. The same holds true for comfort rooms that are used for routine appointments as well. Even euthanasia-only rooms need proper cleaning in between appointments to limit the spread of infectious disease by family members returning home to other pets. This includes wiping down surfaces with disinfectants and vacuuming as needed. As with most procedures, equipment should be cleaned after use. If syringes are to be reused for living patients, they must be sterilized using an autoclave.

## Drugs

The euthanasia drugs we use in everyday practice, whether in the clinic or in the field, are chosen based on (1) availability, (2) cost, (3) reliability and irreversibility, (4) human abuse potential, (5) subsequent use of tissue, (6) carcass disposal, and (7) length of time to death (AVMA euthanasia guidelines draft review 2011). They consist of inhalant gases and noninhalant pharmaceutical agents, both injectable and oral. When pre-euthanasia sedation/anesthesia is required, common sedatives and anesthetics are used.

When the drug in question is Class II-V, they must be kept safe, away from the public, and an accurate drug log maintained. Clinic drug safes or field medicine drug lock boxes must be used to ensure the safety of personnel and eliminate the likelihood of theft. All euthanasia drugs and many pre-euthanasia anesthetics must be locked up and an accurate logging system established. The veterinarian ordering these drugs is required to hold an active veterinary license, a Drug Enforcement Administration (DEA) license, and in some states, hold a Controlled Substance license. However, a DEA license is not required by the attending veterinarian, or "certified euthanasia technicians" typically found in shelters, to perform euthanasia or carry the necessary drugs. Whenever possible, drugs should be kept locked up until the precise time they are needed. Expired and wasted drugs need to be reported to the DEA. Any veterinarian working with large numbers of animals at one time should be prepared to present documentation to DEA enforcement officials in the field if requested. Documentation should include the following:

- The client name
- The patient name or ID
- The species and weight of the animal
- The amount of drug used
- The total amount of the drug left
- The name of the person that administered the drug

## Inhalant agents

> ### Equipment List
>
> *Anesthetic gas examples*: halothane, isoflurane, sevoflurane, and desflurane
> *Gases*: carbon dioxide ($CO_2$), carbon monoxide (CO), nitrogen, and argon

The most suitable inhalant agents are those that rapidly induce unconsciousness before respiratory arrest occurs. A one-size-fits-all approach is impossible to achieve and each animal may require individual protocol adjustments. The following must be considered when choosing an inhaled agent for euthanasia (taken from the (AVMA euthanasia guidelines draft review 2011)):

- Time to unconsciousness depends on many factors.
- The equipment used must be in good working order and legal.
- Most inhaled agents are hazardous to workers.
- Sick or depressed animals may not achieve a timely death.

- Neonatal animals and certain species appear to be resistant to hypoxia.
- Rapid gas flow may produce noise and subsequent aversion.
- Agents are best delivered in a safe environment for the animal.
- Some inhaled agents may be lighter or heavier than air.
- Agents that induce convulsions prior to loss of consciousness are unacceptable.
- Death must be verified before agent exposure is done.

Depending on the gas being delivered to the animal, supplemental oxygen ($O_2$) must be provided to prevent hypoxia before unconsciousness (AVMA euthanasia guidelines draft review 2011).

The AVMA's 2011 guidelines review lists anesthetic gases in order of preferred use as: isoflurane, halothane, sevoflurane, and desflurane. They should be nonirritating to mucous membranes and contain little to no odor. Inhalant agents are typically delivered through facemasks or within chambers, and under rare instances, can be added to water to euthanize fish. The liquid state of most anesthetics is irritating to tissues and should not contact the animal directly. Inhaled anesthetics can be useful as the sole euthanasia agent or as part of a two-step process, where animals are first rendered unconscious through exposure to inhaled anesthetic agents and subsequently euthanized using a secondary method such as intracardiac injection with a pharmaceutical agent, decapitation, etc.

Overdoses of inhalant anesthetics (e.g., ether, halothane, methoxyflurane, isoflurane, sevoflurane, desflurane, enflurane, and nitrous oxide) have been used to euthanize many species (Booth 1988). Those agents not commonly used in private practice are being purposely excluded from this book. Halothane induces anesthesia rapidly and is an effective inhalant agent for euthanasia. Isoflurane is less soluble than halothane, and it induces anesthesia more rapidly. However, it has a pungent odor and onset of unconsciousness may be delayed due to breath holding. Because of lower potency, isoflurane also may require more drug to kill an animal compared with halothane. Sevoflurane is less potent than either isoflurane or halothane and has a lower vapor pressure. Anesthetic concentrations can be achieved and maintained rapidly but more drug will be required to kill the animal. Although sevoflurane is reported to possess less of an objectionable odor than isoflurane, some species may struggle violently and experience apnea when sevoflurane is administered by facemask or induction chamber (Flecknell et al. 1999). Sevoflurane induces epileptiform electrocortical activity, which may be disturbing for onlookers (Voss et al. 2008). Desflurane is currently the least soluble potent inhalant anesthetic, but the vapor is quite pungent, which may slow induction. This drug is so volatile that it could displace $O_2$ and induce hypoxemia during induction if supplemental $O_2$ is not provided. Halothane, isoflurane, sevoflurane, and desflurane are nonflammable and nonexplosive under usual clinical conditions. Precautions should still be taken to limit risk to personnel and animal.

Other inhalant agents include CO, $CO_2$, nitrogen, and argon. They are all considered conditionally acceptable or as adjunctive methods when used with appropriate species. None of them are listed as acceptable methods alone as too many extenuating factors are present. Each gas should be closely understood before use so that delivery is ideal. These gases must be obtained from licensed manufacturers to ensure their purity, concentration, temperature, and delivery rate. Any outside source, including "home creation" is considered unacceptable (AVMA euthanasia guidelines draft review 2011). An example of this would be the use of antacids or dry ice to create $CO_2$ for use in small animals. It is recognized that some gases can be created using alternate sources, but must be delivered at ambient temperatures and purified to remove contaminants prior to exposure (AVMA euthanasia guidelines draft review 2011).

## Noninhalant pharmaceutical agents

As of 2012, within the United States, there are two types of acceptable euthanasia-specific injectable agents: barbiturates and barbiturate combinations (Table 2.2) (AVMA euthanasia guidelines draft review 2011). These agents are widely recognized as "best practice" because they are rapid acting, can be administered in various ways, and have a high percentage of reliability and irreversibility when given properly (Lumb 1974). Pure barbiturates are those containing pentobarbital with no additives and are class II controlled drugs. Typical concentrations range from 260 to 390 mg/mL. Barbiturate-combination drugs include those with phenytoin sodium or lidocaine and are class III controlled drugs due to their lower abuse potential. Powder barbiturates can also be administered orally. Barbiturates are to be kept at room temperature, but remain fairly stable under warmer or colder temperatures.

Other injectable agents, conditionally allowed for use by the World Society for the Protection of Animals (WSPA) and the AVMA include KCl, Tributame®, T-61® (not produced in the United States), and propofol. Others that may be known are not listed here as they are not available within the United States. These four drugs are only acceptable under general anesthesia due to their often unpredictable nature and the risk of distress upon death. They are generally considered unnecessary to use in most animals due to the availability of barbiturates. Some common sedatives such as $\alpha_2$-agonists and dissociatives like ketamine do have lethal doses that can be administered intramuscular (IM) in small animals, but limited study has been conducted on the efficacy of their use and is generally not recommended when other, more predictable agents are available. The AVMA guidelines do list two studies conducted in mice only.

KCl is an adjunctive method in many species. A saturated solution of KCl can be prepared by mixing 560 g KCl in a liter of warm water and stirring. If there is some solid KCl at the bottom of the solution, then the solution is saturated at that temperature. Some people incorrectly refer to this as a supersaturated solution but it is not; it is simply a saturated solution. Methylene blue or some other dye can be added to the solution to help with proper identification.

Other pharmaceutical agents that can be used for euthanasia include many for amphibians and fish. They are ethanol, tricaine methanesulfonate (MS-222), benzocaine hydrochloride, eugenol (clove oil), 2-phenoxyethanol, quinaldine, and metomidate. These agents will be described in more depth within the

**Table 2.2** Injectable euthanasia agents. The IV doses listed are the minimum acceptable amounts for most domestic species. Labels should be consulted to determine appropriate usage in various species.

| Pentobarbital sodium | Class II | |
| --- | --- | --- |
| **Name** | **Concentration** | **IV dose** |
| Fatal Plus® | 390 mg/mL | 1 mL per 10 lbs |
| Socumb-6gr® | Same as above | |
| Somlethol® | Same as above | |
| Sleepaway® | 260 mg/mL | |
| Pentobarbital sodium with Phenytoin sodium | Class III | |
| **Name** | **Concentration** | **Dose** |
| Beuthanasia-D | 390 mg/mL (pentobarb) | 1 mL per10 lbs |
| | 50 mg/mL (phenytoin) | |
| Euthasol® | Same as above | |
| Euthanasia-III® | Same as above | |
| Pentobarbital sodium with lidocaine | Class III | |
| **Name** | **Concentration** | **Dose** |
| FP-3®ᵃ | 390 mg/mL (pentobarb) | 1 mL per 10 lbs |
| | 20 mg/mL (lidocaine) | |
| Secobarbitol sodium with dibucaine | Class III | |
| **Name** | **Concentration** | **Dose** |
| Repose®ᵃ | 400 mg/mL (secobarbitol) | 0.22 mL/kg |
| | 25 mg/mL (dibucaine) | |
| Embutramide | Class III | |
| **Name** | **Concentration** | **Dose** |
| T-61ᵃ | 200 mg/mL (embutramide) | 0.14 mL/lb |
| | 50 mg/mL (mebozonium iodide) | |
| | 5 mg/mL (tetracaine HCl) | |
| Tributameᵃ | 135 mg/mL (embutramide) | 1 mL per 5 lb |
| | 35 mg/mL (chloroquine phosphate) | |
| | 1.9 mg/mL (lidocaine) | |
| Potassium chloride (KCl) | | |
| **Name** | **Concentration** | **Dose** |
| KCl | Varies | 1-2 mmol/kg |

ᵃThese products are currently marketed in the United States.

**Table 2.3** Common pre-euthanasia drugs.

| Dissociatives | Class | Common names |
|---|---|---|
| Tiletamine/zolazepam | III | Telazol® |
| Ketamine | III | Ketaset®, Ketaved® |
| $\alpha_2$-agonists | | |
| Xylazine | - | Rompun®, Ketased® Anased® |
| Medetomidine | - | Domitor® |
| Dexmedetomidine | - | Dexdomitor® |
| Opiates | | |
| Butorphanol | IV | Torbugesic® Dolorex® |
| Buprenorphine | III | Buprenex® |
| Morphine | II | none |
| Nalbuphine | - | none |
| Fentanyl | II | Fentanyl® |
| Phenothiazines | | |
| Acepromazine | - | PromAce® |
| Benzodiazepines | | |
| Diazepam | IV | Valium® |
| Midazelam | IV | Midazelam |

exotic's technique section in Chapter 5. Agents, such as formaldehyde, that are rarely used in private practice will not be discussed in any great detail.

## Pre-euthanasia drugs

When sedation is needed, such as with a fractious animal or when the clinic's policy is pre-euthanasia sedation/anesthesia for every pet, a variety of pre-euthanasia sedatives and anesthetics need to be kept on location along with the euthanasia drug of choice (Table 2.3). Each drug's method of action, metabolism, etc., needs to be fully understood before use. Most may be given IV, IM, or subcutaneous (SQ), and some may be given orally to induce sedation. When given orally, some can be squirted directly into the mouth or canned food must be kept on site to mix with. More on all of these drugs and their role in euthanasia will be discussed in Chapter 4.

## Species-specific considerations

## Dogs and cats

The euthanasia of dogs and cats is usually accomplished by the IV administration of noninhalant pharmaceutical agents such as pentobarbital. Restraint devices such as muzzles, cat bags, and squeeze cages may be needed to hold the animal prior to euthanasia. Because the cats and dogs that veterinarians encounter, particularly dogs, come in a variety of sizes, needles and syringes

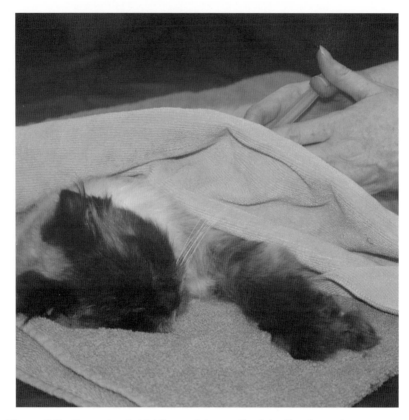

**Figure 2.8** Example of shielding an intracardiac injection from view.

of various sizes should be on hand. For most dogs and cats, syringes ranging in size from 3 to 20 mL will be adequate. Normal needle sizes used for administering pre-euthanasia sedation/anesthesia and euthanasia solution range from 25 to 18 gauge with a typical length of 0.5–1 in.

When families are present or when the pet is not sedated, ideal circumstances will have the veterinarian placing an IV catheter (AVMA euthanasia guidelines draft review 2011). Catheters used typically range from 25 to 20 gauge. Tape can be used to anchor the setup to the leg. When necessary, bandage scissors and hemostats may be needed to remove firmly placed catheter setups from the leg.

When venous access is not possible, longer needles up to 3 in. in length may be needed to perform an intracardiac or deep organ injection. If watching a technique like this is difficult for the client, a small cloth drape can be used to shield the injection from view (Figure 2.8). Longer needles may also be required to reach the liver in large dogs.

Euthanasia via gunshot is the only conditionally acceptable physical method for use on dogs and cats (AVMA euthanasia guidelines draft review 2011). Within 3 ft of the animal, the gun must be of the appropriate caliber, usually no larger than a .22 handgun or rifle. If the distance is greater, such as within 5–15 yards, a shotgun of 12, 16, or 20 gauge, with #6 to #2 shot may be used

(AWIC 2002). The use of gunshot is not allowed for routine use and should only be attempted when no other humane method is available and the animal is suffering.

The use of inhalant agents such as anesthetic gases, CO, and $CO_2$ for dog and cat euthanasia are generally considered conditionally acceptable, meaning multiple factors must be met for their use. Anesthetic gases may be delivered via intubation tubes during surgery or via gas mask. CO and $CO_2$ may be delivered via closely monitored chambers. Nitrogen and Argon are utilized only as adjunctive methods when no other technique is available and the pet is already rendered unconscious.

## Exotics

Equipment necessary for most small companion exotics and birds that a veterinarian will encounter in a hospital setting is minimal. When using injectable agents, an assortment of small needles ranging from 27 to 20 gauge should be available with lengths ranging from 0.5 to 2 in. Syringe sizes are those similar to dogs and cats.

For inhalant gas use, a closed container must be used, such as an anesthetic mask sized appropriately to fit the patient. Plastic bottles work well with waterfowl and wading birds to fit their long beaks. A latex glove can be placed over the large opening and a hole cut in to place the beak through. Other various containers include plastic tubes for snakes or plastic bags to fit over the patient's face. A plastic shoebox for guinea pigs or rabbits can be used for gas anesthetic induction or euthanasia, and the smallest possible container will help the process go faster.

When using immersion solutions to achieve euthanasia in amphibians and fish, an appropriate reservoir, such as a leak-proof pan or tank, will be needed. The animal will be placed in the solution for topical or inhalant absorption. Gloves should be worn to prevent uptake through the administrator's skin and a lid should be placed over the top of the reservoir to prevent escape.

Physical methods, such as decapitation of small rodents, birds, reptiles, and amphibians, will require a sharp cutting tool to efficiently sever the head from the neck. Pre-euthanasia anesthesia will be required unless the animal is already unconscious. Rapid freezing with liquid nitrogen is conditionally acceptable for those <4 kg.

For assistance in handling the patients, a variety of towels should be available for use. Sacks such as pillowcases work well for containing snakes prior to handling and thick leather gloves are helpful for handling raptors and sharp-scaled animals such as iguanas.

Pet crocodilians and other large reptiles can be euthanized by a penetrating captive bolt or gunshot (free bullet) delivered to the brain (Made 1996). Decapitation of small rodents, birds, and reptiles can be completed using a sharp blade or shears.

A doplar unit and small stethoscope accurate enough to auscult small patients is very helpful for accurate assessment of cardiac arrest (Figures 2.9 and 2.10).

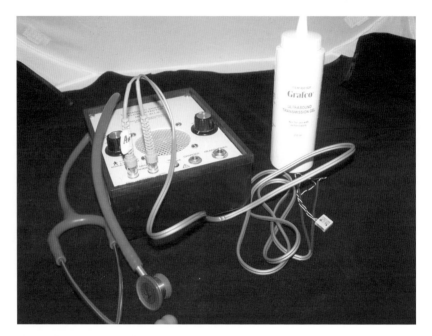

**Figure 2.9** Common doplar unit.

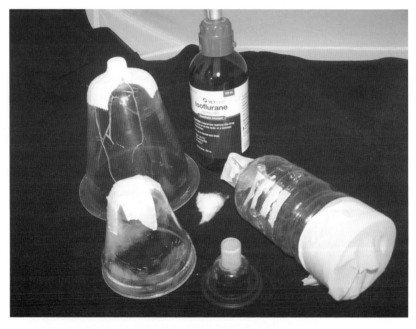

**Figure 2.10** Masks modified for very small animals.

## Horses

Horses, mules, and donkeys can be euthanized using noninhalant injectable agents and physical methods. Due to their size, the use of inhalant euthanasia agents is almost never attempted. None of the drugs or instruments used for equine euthanasia are unique from other species, but there are unique ways they can be utilized.

Veterinarians should use their best judgment as to the best equipment to use with horses. If restraint is needed, a halter and lead rope is usually sufficient for nonfractious horses. Towels can be used to cover the eyes to help quiet an anxious horse. If necessary, a squeeze chute can be used to hold the horse in place, but once the euthanasia is complete, it can be difficult to remove them from the area. A rodeo roughstock chute could be acceptable as could a livestock alley. It should be noted that squeeze chutes can be extremely dangerous for horses and for the people working around them. The chute engenders claustrophobic panic and extreme attempts to escape.

IV barbiturates are probably the most widely used method of equine euthanasia in the United States, followed by gunshot and penetrating captive bolt. Barbiturates are almost always administered in the jugular vein along the lateral side of the neck. Due to the large size of the horse, a high volume of euthanasia solution must be administered and done so as quickly as possible. Large bore needles, such as the 16–14-gauge, 2-in. size are commonly used for direct venipuncture into the jugular vein. If venous pressures are very poor and the veins are difficult to feel, such as with a sick foal, an intracardiac injection can be performed using a large bore 4–6-in. needle. When catheters are used, a minimum of a 16-gauge size is recommended with attached 3-mL extension set. When using a high-viscosity euthanasia solution such as Beuthanasia-D®, the added length of the extension set can make pushing the solution difficult. Syringe size is also important. Larger syringes hold more solution and should to used to administer as fast as possible.

When attempting a physical method such as the gunshot at close range, pistols such as the .22 LR caliber or .380 caliber can be used on small horses or foals. A larger caliber pistol will allow the veterinarian more leeway in placement if needed. The use of a hollow point bullet will maximize tissue damage and decrease the possibility of ricochet.

If the horse cannot be manually restrained, a gunshot must be attempted from a distance. A rifle or shotgun may be used, but the excessive power may increase the risk of the bullet passing through the horse and into the environment. Great care must be taken when this is attempted.

The captive bolt technique uses the same types of bolt guns as used with other species. When required to use a physical method in an urban setting, the bolt gun should replace the use of gun and ammunition. It is considered safer than gunshot.

Emergency situations may arise where there is no access to any of the aforementioned equipment. In young foals, a blow to the head may be effective, but it must penetrate the skull and disrupt the brain to effect immediate humane euthanasia. A strong pointed instrument such as a miner's pick or fireman's pick axe could be used with effect similar to captive bolt, but will require a skilled operator to be humane. This technique would be much more difficult to perform on an adult horse. The combination of stunning the animal with a blow to the head followed by exsanguination is effective, but also technically difficult. Exsanguination may be carried out using a 6-in. blade across the throatlatch or per rectum to transect the aorta using any blade equal to or larger than a scalpel blade.

## Livestock

Livestock veterinarians should be prepared for the possible need to perform euthanasia on any farm call. In some cases, the potential for euthanasia is clear from the client's request at the time of making the appointment, or based on the presenting complaint for the visit. However, it is possible that the information received prior to the appointment may not indicate that euthanasia may be necessary. For routine farm calls, there is always the possibility for unforeseen accidents or complications that may necessitate euthanizing an animal. For example, one does not expect to have to euthanize an animal while performing routine herd vaccinations or pregnancy examinations. However, there is always risk associated with chutes, equipment, and procedures that could result in fractures, back or spinal injury, head trauma, neck injury, or other complications that are not readily treatable and may result in euthanasia of the animal. For these reasons, it is recommended that euthanasia supplies be considered part of the standard equipment available for all farm calls.

Even though many different species are considered livestock, most of the same supplies can be used among them. As with the other domesticated animals discussed, IV administration of a barbiturate is common practice with livestock, except for those intended for food. Syringe sizes vary and are based on the size of the animal being helped. As with all species, the bigger the animal, the bigger the syringe needed. Needle sizes range from 20 to 18 gauge × 1.5 in. for small ruminants or camelids to 14 gauge × 2 in. for adult cattle. If an IV catheter must be placed, 18–16 gauge up to 3 in. is ideal for small ruminants or camelids. Larger livestock do well with 16–14-gauge × 3-5-in. catheters.

A .22-caliber firearm, when used appropriately will reliably render most livestock immediately unconscious with a single appropriately placed shot. Soft or hollow point .22-caliber bullets may be used in calves, sheep, or goats and will reduce the risk of the bullet exiting the target. Soft or hollow point .22-caliber bullets may not penetrate the skull of adult cattle and are not recommended. A .22-caliber long rifle solid point (round nose) bullet is better suited for adult cattle and swine but may still lack the energy to penetrate large cows, bulls, or boars.

Adequate projectile energy and penetration is more likely when using a rifle compared to a pistol. A .22 magnum cartridge is generally sufficient for cattle >24 months of age but many veterinarians still prefer a higher caliber firearm. It must be noted that in some cases, standard .22 or .22 magnum caliber firearms may not result in sufficient cerebral trauma to cause cardiac or respiratory arrest, particularly in large adult cattle and swine. Thus, secondary methods of inducing cardiac and respiratory arrest should be available such as pithing, exsanguination, IV KCl, or pneumothorax.

Some states may set specific standards for livestock euthanasia by firearm. For example, the Ohio Livestock Care Standards Board specifically requires a .22 long rifle or larger caliber hollow point cartridge for small livestock and immature cattle or swine, and a minimum .22 magnum hollow point for mature cattle and swine (Ohio Livestock Care Standards Board, http://ohiolivestockcarestandardsboard.gov/content/news/effective_standards.aspx).

For mature bulls and boars, a 9-mm, .357-caliber, or larger, firearm is recommended. If you are relying on the firearm to render the animal both unconscious and inflict enough central nervous system (CNS) damage to result in cardiac and respiratory arrest, then a .44 magnum should be used. Hollow or soft point bullets should be considered for 9-mm or larger rounds to minimize the risk of the projectile exiting the animal and possibly causing human injury or property damage. This is particularly a concern when using a large caliber firearm for small ruminants or calves. A 12-gauge shotgun is recommended for larger livestock such as bulls or boars.

There is no single firearm and bullet that is optimum for all classes of livestock (Table 2.1). Both .22-caliber pistols and rifles are satisfactory for most species and age of livestock. A .22-caliber survival rifle is a light, compact, low-cost, and durable firearm for the ambulatory setting, but has been known to cause ricochet when striking a hard object at an angle. Some studies have shown that a ricocheted .22-caliber bullet can travel up to 0.5 mile. A hunting rifle with a telescopic scope may be the best alternative in situations where you cannot approach the animal for euthanasia at close range. In the end, the selection of the firearm is determined by local regulations, the appropriate ballistics needed for the animal to be euthanized, and personal preference.

Both penetrating and nonpenetrating captive bolt stunners are available for euthanasia of livestock. The nonpenetrating captive bolt device has a mushroom head and stuns the animal solely by concussive force. In general, the nonpenetrating captive bolt stunner is not considered a reliable method for field euthanasia of livestock. Along with the concussive impact to the skull, penetrating captive bolt stunners cause additional irreversible physical trauma to the brain, including portions of the cerebrum, midbrain, pons, cerebellum, and medulla oblongata depending on method. Penetration and physical trauma to the brain will cause irreversible loss of consciousness provided the appropriate areas are destroyed. For this reason, the penetrating captive bolt stunner is generally preferred for veterinary euthanasia (Tables 2.4 and 2.5).

**Table 2.4** Trigger fire captive bolt stunners (models available in 2011).

| Model | Caliber | Bolt length | Recommended species |
|---|---|---|---|
| Cash Special Accles & Shelvoke | .22 and .25 | 121 mm (4 3/4 inch) | Sheep, swine, cattle |
| Cash Magnum Accles & Shelvoke | .22 and .25 | 121 mm (4 3/4 inch) | Cattle |
| Cash Special Heavy Duty Accles & Shelvoke | .25 | 121 mm (4 3/4 inch) | Cattle |
| Cash Special HD Extended Bolt Accles & Shelvoke | .25 | 136 mm (5 3/8 inch) | Large cattle |
| Cash Dispatch Kit Accles & Shelvoke | .25 | Variable | Poultry, swine, sheep, horses, neonates, and adult |
| Blitz-Kerner Captive Bolt Stunner | 9 mm | 57 mm (2 1/4 inch) | Growing swine, gilts, sheep, calves, light cattle |
| Schermer KR Stunner | NA | 82 mm (3 1/4 inch) | Sheep, swine, cattle |
| Schermer KC Non-Penetrating Stunner | NA | 82 mm (3 1/4 inch) | Sheep, swine, cattle |
| Schermer KS Self-Retracting Stunner | NA | 82 mm (3 1/4 inch) | Sheep, swine, cattle |
| Schermer KL Stunner Elongated Bolt | NA | 133 mm (5 1/4 inch) | Cattle |

**Table 2.5** Captive Bolt Stunner manufacturers and US distributors.

| Manufacturers | Website |
|---|---|
| Accles & Shelvoke, West Midlands, England | www.acclesandshelvoke.co.uk/index.htm |
| Karl Schermer Gmbh & Co., Ettlingen, Germany | www.karl-schermer.de |
| **US Distributors** | |
| Bunzl Processor Division (Koch Supplies), North Kansas City, MO | www.bunzlprocessor.com |
| Cotran Corporation, Portsmout, RI | www.cotrancorp.com |
| Hantover, Kansas City, MO | www.hantover.com |
| Hog Slat Inc., Newton Grove, NC | http://hogslat.biz/Blitz_Captive_Bolt_Stunner.asp |
| QC Supply, Schuyler, NE | www.qcsupply.com/farm-livestock/handling/bolt-stunners.html |
| AGRIsales Inc., Ceresco, NE | http://www.agrisales-inc.com |

# Chapter 3
# Positioning and Restraint

It is well agreed upon by the veterinary and animal professional community that the more comfortable and relaxed the animal, the smoother the euthanasia process. As we have been discussing so far, the key to euthanasia is to provide a pain-free, anxiety-free death for each animal. It is difficult to know exactly what an animal understands about the position it is placed in, but we do know that keeping it in familiar surroundings will lessen stress. An ideal euthanasia setting for a client-owned dog or cat might include loved ones gathered around, remaining at home on its bed, or within a safe setting at the hospital, while an ideal setting for a fractious stray might be minimal human contact, kept in a quiet dimly lit room, and given a pre-euthanasia sedative before handling. Horses and livestock do best in areas where they have been safely handled before, and so on. Regardless of the temperament, all animals should be treated with love and compassion before and after euthanasia.

All personnel performing euthanasia must be well educated in animal behavior and husbandry. Education is paramount to assuring that the animal's body language is understood. For example, if the handler witnesses a display of fear, the animal cannot be guaranteed a distress-free death. It is also important for euthanasia personnel to understand the normal anatomy for the animal, the limitations of the physical body, for example, range of limb motion, head extension, and so on. Excessive restraint can make the situation worse. Salivation, vocalization, urination, defecation, evacuation of anal sacs, pupillary dilatation, tachycardia, sweating, and reflex skeletal muscle contractions causing shivering, tremors, or other muscular spasms may occur in unconscious as well as conscious animals (AVMA euthanasia guidelines draft review 2011). Readers are encouraged to increase their understanding of animal behavior for the benefit of the animal and their own safety.

## Positioning

Positioning is dependent on the euthanasia technique being performed, the use of pre-euthanasia sedatives, and the species being aided. As will be

*Veterinary Euthanasia Techniques: A Practical Guide*, First Edition. Kathleen A. Cooney, Jolynn R. Chappell, Robert J. Callan and Bruce A. Connally.
© 2012 John Wiley & Sons, Inc. Published 2012 by John Wiley & Sons, Inc.

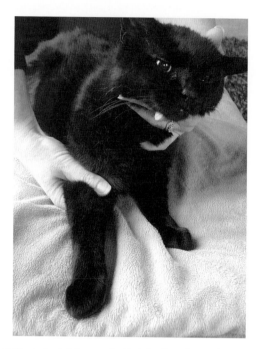

**Figure 3.1**   Gentle restraint for cephalic injection in a cat.

discussed in Chapter 5, animals have to be positioned appropriately for the particular technique being utilized. Those being euthanized with injectable agents will be handled differently than those exposed to inhalants, etc. Depending on the location, small animals may be euthanized on the table, on the floor, on the client's lap, and so on. Larger animals may be euthanized in stalls, in stocks, out in pasture, and so on. When family is involved, small animals may be held as long as the person holding is protected from scratching and biting. Many veterinarians have service policies against families holding pets to avoid injury and subsequent lawsuits, especially those working with large animals.

Positioning and necessary restraint will depend a lot on the temperament of the animal. Proper restraining techniques will minimize distress for all animals, regardless of their exposure and comfort with humans. In the case of companion animals, those that are familiar with human love and protection do well with gentle touches, soft voices, and support from their family. If the pet is fearful of people, such as in the case of abused or feral animals, or is extremely painful, minimal contact is preferred. Those present will need to determine what is best for the animal and themselves given the situation (Figure 3.1).

Regardless of the method of euthanasia, the animal must be clearly visible and safe to handle. For example, proper lighting is important so that the injection site can be easily seen. In situations where light is minimized, such as outdoor evening appointments or clinic power outages, flashlights should be used. Every hospital should have backup light sources in the case of such an event during euthanasia. The animal must be positioned to allow easy visibility and access to the anatomical area of interest.

## Restraint

Restraint can be physical, chemical, or both. The level of restraint needed is based on the method of euthanasia being performed, the temperament of the animal, and experience of the handler, and is used to keep the pet in proper position. The use of restraint does not imply that the animal is fractious. Gentle restraint is typically done with even the calmest animal to ensure that they do not move during an injection, etc. However, if an unsedated animal moves during the euthanasia procedure, it may experience pain and distress. For this reason, many veterinarians are moving toward using pre-euthanasia sedation/anesthesia for all euthanasia procedures. This is considered chemical restraint and can aid the veterinarian in many ways. More on this will be discussed in Chapter 4.

There are numerous ways to restrain an animal for euthanasia. A great description of restraint techniques for small animals can be found in *The HSUS Euthanasia Training Manual* by Rebecca Rhoades, DVM. This manual goes into nice detail regarding cat and dog restraint in particular. The best method is one that feels natural to the animal. It is always important to remember that as comfortable as the restraint hold might be to the animal, it may move very quickly to seek escape. The handler must be prepared for this and respond accordingly to keep everyone safe.

Restraint devices should be kept anywhere animals will be euthanized. Something as simple as a towel can be utilized to gently restrain a dog, cat, or an exotic or can be used to cover the eyes of livestock, etc. Other devices such as muzzles, cat bags, squeeze cages, and gloves limit the risk to personnel and aim to speed the process along for the animal while minimizing human contact. More on restraint will be included below.

In general, regardless of the technique being performed or the temperament of the animal, positioning and the amount of restraint used should be determined on an individual basis. Those with the most experience should be enlisted to assist the person performing the euthanasia. If restraint and proper positioning is proving difficult, pre-euthanasia sedation should be used sooner than later for the comfort of the pet and safety to those handling it.

## Species-specific considerations

### Dogs and cats

In the clinic setting, positioning of the pet will be determined in large part by where the euthanasia is conducted. In the typical examination room, dogs and cats are commonly placed on the examination table, either directly on its

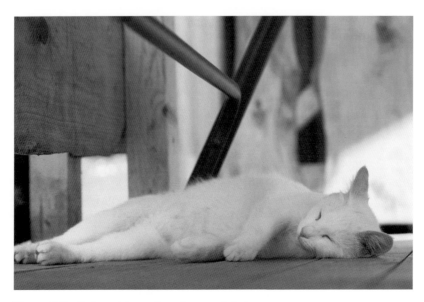

**Figure 3.2** Calm cat free of environmental stressors.

surface or on top of a towel/blanket. Providing a nonslip surface may help the pet feel more secure. A larger dog may be euthanized on the floor to avoid lifting. Many clinics provide floor mats for improved comfort. When hospital space allows, a "comfort" room should be established for easier work with the pet and those gathered around. There is generally more room to position the pet comfortably while allowing the family to gather close. Euthanasia is occasionally conducted during a surgical operation when it is discovered that postsurgery suffering is imminent. When this occurs, the pet may remain in its surgical position or be moved to allow for the best euthanasia technique given the pet's condition.

In the home setting, there are usually more factors affecting the pet's positioning: confinement in a small space, on the master bed, outside on a hillside, and so on. Families choosing home euthanasia appreciate the attending veterinarian's flexibility in accommodating their wishes (Cooney 2011). Every effort should be made to keep the pet comfortable while still performing a technically proficient euthanasia.

If restraint is needed beyond simple holding, a more fractious pet can be immobilized using large blankets, squeeze cages, and so on. Muzzles and cat bags can be used on those pets that will allow it. Ideally, chemical restraint can be offered to calm the dog or cat and keep the handler safe. If none are available, the euthanasia should be carried out as quickly as possible to avoid distress carrying on longer than necessary (Figure 3.2).

## Exotics

Handlers will need to be well versed in exotic handling techniques before attempting euthanasia. For example, some exotics like ferrets are difficult to restrain with towels due to the amount of wriggling they commonly attempt. Handling rabbits properly will decrease their stress level and keep them safer. Protecting their back from injury is essential. Rabbits have powerful hind legs that can kick out and cause injury to themselves or the handler. To prevent this, it is helpful to wrap their body firmly with a towel, and then pick them up, supporting their hind end and cradling their body against the handler's body. Keeping a firm hold on them with their eyes covered usually keeps them calm. Unless the rabbit is quite debilitated, some form of sedation is preferred prior to euthanasia to decrease the stress level, as most rabbits are quite stressed being handled. Most birds can be restrained using towels. Birds of prey can also be hooded to prevent stress.

For guinea pigs, chinchillas, rats, and other pocket pets, they generally do not respond well to handling. Quite commonly, they are very debilitated upon presentation, and when handled, can become quite agitated. The handler can scruff the rodents by placing a hand over the dorsal aspect of the neck and picking up a large handful of skin. Hamsters' eyes tend to become exopthalmic when too much force is applied to their bodies and can even dislodge from the sockets. This can be prevented by placing gentle pressure over the eyes. For more information on handling exotics, there are numerous books devoted to the subject.

## Horses

The actual process of euthanizing a horse, donkey, or mule needs to be orchestrated with safety for the people and humane treatment for the patient as the top two priorities. If this is an emergency euthanasia in a public setting, call the appropriate law enforcement authority. They can assist with crowd and traffic control to keep people safe.

The equine patient needs to be moved away from other animals, as they may present a distraction. Distractions often translate into safety issues. The client may request that they be allowed to hold the horse. Many veterinarians, including this author, discourage this. The client is often dealing with profound grief, which makes them less effective at restraining the horse and less responsive in keeping themselves safe. It is preferable to have a trained technician restrain the animal for practical reasons and for the legal liability as a veterinarian.

It is important to emphasize to all involved that the horse's response to barbiturate euthanasia may be unpredictable. They may sink quietly to the ground but may also fall over backward or lunge forward putting even an experienced horse handler at risk. In some cases, especially when using a firearm, the procedure may be performed without an assistant to minimize risk for those involved.

Physical restraints such as stocks are rarely used due to the difficulty of extricating the body afterward. Any confined space, including stalls or horse trailers, increases the risk for the people involved because the avenues for escape are limited. Veterinarians and those assisting are advised to think through all possible outcomes before attempting equine euthanasia.

## Livestock

Both positioning and restraint of the animal will aid in accomplishing a successful euthanasia. For the primary methods of euthanasia described in this book, access to either the head or neck, or both, is required. This can be attained in both standing and recumbent animals. For large livestock, one should also consider the location of the animal at the time of euthanasia and how that relates to removal or disposal of the carcass. For obvious reasons, large livestock should not be euthanized in a chute or narrow alleyway unless there is a way of opening the side to remove the carcass.

Adequate restraint is essential for a safe and efficient euthanasia in livestock. This may come in the form of chemical restraint, physical restraint, or a combination of both. The key guiding principle is to provide sufficient restraint to minimize stress, discomfort, or pain associated with the procedure. In practical terms, this implies sufficient restraint to either perform a competent venipuncture, or sufficiently stabilize the head for an accurate gunshot or captive bolt stun. The safety of the operator, handlers, and bystanders is also a concern and is optimized with proper restraint of the patient.

Except for very docile or obtunded animals, some degree of physical restraint is helpful and often required to stabilize the head and neck and provide safety. For manageable adult cattle and calves, a halter may be all that is needed to stabilize the head for gunshot or captive bolt stunning. This can be secured to a stable post or other sturdy object, or in some instances held by an assistant. When an assistant holds the halter, they should be positioned to the side and behind the person firing the gun or captive bolt stunner if possible to minimize risk of injury from the projectile or the animal. Sometimes, using two halters and cross-tying the animal will provide more restraint of the head and improve accuracy of the shot. In recumbent cattle, a single halter can be placed, pulling the head to the side and securing the lead around the rear leg and tied at the level of the stifle to provide stabilization of the head and neck. This will provide good restraint allowing for either direct venipuncture and lethal injection or euthanasia by gunshot or stunning.

Simple restraint with a halter may not be sufficient for many cattle, particularly beef cattle. These animals may need to be restrained in an alleyway or a head chute to either allow for injectable sedation or direct euthanasia. If euthanizing an animal in a head chute, one must first consider how the animal will be removed from the chute. This generally requires a chute that has the ability to open or remove at least one side of the chute. In this case, it is very important to release the side gate before euthanizing the animal. Otherwise, when the animal becomes recumbent, it can put so much pressure on the sides of the chute that the chute side cannot be released and opened (Figure 3.3).

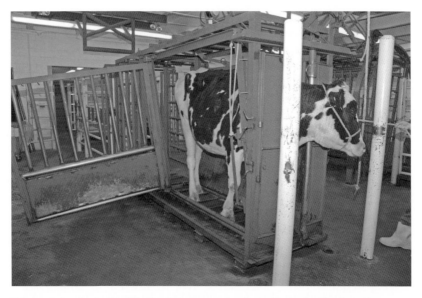

**Figure 3.3** A chute with the side open prior to euthanasia. The head is restrained with a halter and would allow for safe euthanasia by intravenous injection, gunshot, or captive bolt stunning. The head is pulled slightly to the animal's left so that the animal will fall to the right side.

The mechanics of euthanasia in sheep and goats is generally the same as in cattle except that the animals are smaller and more easily restrained. As with cattle, the goal is to position the animal so that the head and neck are accessible for either intravenous (IV) injection or euthanasia by physical means such as gunshot or captive bolt. For severely ill, obtunded, or recumbent animals, only minimal physical restraint may be necessary. Even in alert and active animals, gentle physical restraint is often sufficient. A halter can also be used. A head catch or chute is rarely necessary to restrain a sheep or goat for euthanasia. Access to the jugular veins for IV injection can be obtained with the animal standing or in sternal recumbency and the head bent slightly away from the side of the injection. Alternatively, the animal can be positioned in lateral recumbency.

Euthanasia of swine can be more challenging than other livestock species due to the difficulty of proper restraint and positioning. In general, pigs do not accept physical restraint. In severely debilitated or obtunded animals, this may not be an issue. However, many times, the pigs are sufficiently active enough to struggle when restrained. This can make humane euthanasia by lethal injection particularly challenging. While pig snares can be used, this often results in significant resistance and distress in the pig. Another alternative for smaller pigs is to restrain the pig suspended in a sling. This may allow access to the cephalic vein for IV injection. However, because of the challenges with restraint and venipuncture, humane euthanasia performed by lethal injection may be best performed following heavy sedation or anesthesia to allow for a calm venipuncture or intracardiac injection. Otherwise, gunshot or captive bolt methods should be utilized.

Like the other livestock species, euthanasia of llamas and alpacas requires adequate restraint that allows access to the head and jugular vein. Many llamas and alpacas are sufficiently manageable to be restrained simply with a halter and lead rope. Unmanageable animals may need further restraint with either a camelid chute or sedation. Llamas, with their larger size, can be difficult to satisfactorily restrain on lead if they have not previously been worked with.

Sometimes, just catching the llama or alpaca can be a challenge, particularly if they are in a large field or pen. In those cases, a long rope held between two or more people can help corral the animal into a corner and allow them to be haltered. As with the other species, many of the animals that require euthanasia are debilitated and may not have the strength to object to basic physical restraint.

Sedation may be appropriate in some cases, particularly when simple physical restraint is not sufficient, or if the owner specifically requests it. The primary reason for using sedation would be if the animal cannot be restrained sufficiently to allow for proficient jugular venipuncture, or an accurate gunshot or captive bolt stun. The same sedatives that are used in ruminants can also be used in llamas and alpacas, although they tend to require higher doses.

# Chapter 4
# Pre-euthanasia Sedation and Anesthesia

When we think about assisting an animal with euthanasia, the terms "peaceful" and "painfree" hopefully come to mind. There are many factors to consider when preparing to help an animal achieve a good death. How can we make it as pain free as possible? How can we reduce stress? Will it be quick? The whole premise behind euthanasia is to help the animal die in as comfortable a manner as possible, and pre-euthanasia sedation or anesthesia is a great way to facilitate that. This being said, it must still be recognized that sedatives or anesthetics may delay the onset of the euthanasia agent (AVMA euthanasia guidelines draft review 2011).

There is a distinct difference between simple sedation and anesthesia; however the terms are commonly interchanged. The American Veterinary Medical Association (AVMA) guidelines indicate that general anesthesia or unconsciousness is required for some conditionally acceptable or adjunctive methods. This means that the animal in question must be given enough anesthetic agent to induce unconsciousness and prevent pain perception. Sedation, on the other hand, indicates that while the animal may be relaxed and free of mild to moderate pain, it is revivable and may become distressed if enough painful stimuli is applied.

Generalizations may be made as to what type of drug works well for a particular age, disease, or physical attribute an animal may possess, but it is up to the attending veterinarian to modify the protocol as needed. Understanding the drug's mode of action, common side effects, etc., will help ensure that the animal remains comfortable and stable throughout the procedure.

There will be times when administering an anesthetic agent to a pet is more distressing than performing the euthanasia itself. An example of this is the small fractious pet that must be restrained for an anesthetic injection when an intraperitoneal (IP) injection of a barbiturate would be just as effective. The use for and against pre-euthanasia sedation/anesthesia must be based on the

*Veterinary Euthanasia Techniques: A Practical Guide*, First Edition. Kathleen A. Cooney, Jolynn R. Chappell, Robert J. Callan and Bruce A. Connally.
© 2012 John Wiley & Sons, Inc. Published 2012 by John Wiley & Sons, Inc.

> ## Box 4.1 Reasons for and against pre-euthanasia sedation or anesthesia in domestic animals
>
> ### Pros
> Minimizes distress for the animal
> Eliminates pre-death pain from the animal's disease
> Lessens danger to the handlers
> Increases technique options
> Eliminates need for restraint during euthanasia
> Eliminates need for second person to assist
> May lessen perimortem side effects, for example, agonal breathing
>
> ### Cons
> More expensive
> May alter body physiology making certain techniques more difficult
> Unpredictable transition into sedation with critical patients
> Potential for side effects, for example, vomiting, dyspnea

pet being euthanized, the skill of the handler, and the method of euthanasia itself.

## Anesthesia

There are varying levels of anesthesia, but the AVMA is generally referring to surgical-depth anesthesia. The guidelines are written this way in direct response to scientific study indicating that pain will be felt by a particular method unless unconsciousness is achieved. General anesthesia will be required for those conditionally acceptable methods where pain and distress are a probability in a conscious animal, such as intracardiac (IC) injections with a noninhalant pharmaceutical agent, electrocution, or potassium chloride (KCl) administration.

Following are the four stages of anesthesia (Rhoades 2002):

(1) *Voluntary excitement*: The pet is hypersensitive to noise and touch while losing consciousness. Gentle touch and a quiet presence are important.
(2) *Involuntary excitement*: This is considered an unpredictable time. If held too long in this stage, the pet may be disorientated, vocalize, bite, leg paddle, and move sporadically.
(3) *Anesthesia*: This is considered a surgical level of anesthesia with the pet unconscious, and in its deepest phase, and has no response to internal or external stimuli. Vital functions remain intact and are considered easily reversible.

(4) *Medullary paralysis*: This happens when the surgical plane of anesthesia becomes too deep and the pet is overdosing. It is life threatening. Respiratory and cardiac arrest are the end results of fatal medullary paralysis.[1]

The administration of anesthetic agents should move the animal gently through the first three stages. Many can be given orally, by injection, or through inhalation and can be done in a one- or two-step protocol. When the method of euthanasia is injection through an intravenous (IV) catheter with an agent like pentobarbital, some veterinarians will perform a one-step anesthetic protocol with an anesthetic drug immediately preceding the fatal injection. This is similar to an anesthetic inhalant being offered before euthanasia. Some veterinarians will administer a pre-euthanasia sedative to effect, and then follow it with a true anesthetic agent just before proceeding with euthanasia. This is considered a two-step pre-euthanasia anesthesia protocol. This protocol helps ensure that the animal will not experience any physical change between sedation and death.

For euthanasia itself, using an inhalant or noninhalant pharmaceutical agent, the animal should move smoothly through all four stages of anesthesia to achieve cardiac death. Barbiturates such as pentobarbital are effectively an anesthetic overdose with the intent to reach stage four as rapidly as possible. They can be, and were commonly used before, as anesthetic drugs themselves. Other anesthetic injectable agents such as propofol can also be used to facilitate euthanasia by way of anesthetic overdose.

## Sedation

Sedation is a term used to describe a light state of anesthesia wherein the pet is generally unaware of its surroundings but remains responsive to painful stimulation (Tranquilli and Thurmon 2007). This means that the pet's ability to react normally to its environment is altered, but it generally does not go to the point of unconsciousness with absolutely zero ability to respond to stimuli such as pain, noise, or light. Sedation can be achieved by administering sedative drugs at therapeutic doses or by administering true anesthetic drugs below levels required for surgical anesthesia.

The decision of whether or not to sedate an animal prior to euthanasia is a very personal choice and is reflected by an individual's previous training, experience, and the circumstances of the specific euthanasia. Sedation of the animal may be requested by the client or the person performing the euthanasia may determine that sedation of the animal would make the procedure less aversive to onlookers (Figure 4.1). Some individuals feel that sedation decreases the risk of excitatory or violent responses by the animal during or

[1]Some literature create a Stage 5 for cardiac death.

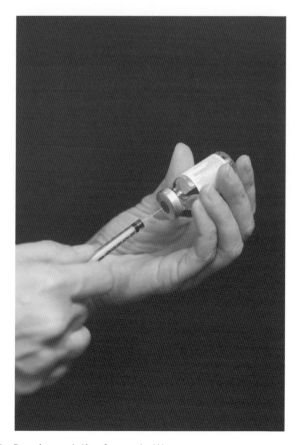

**Figure 4.1**   Drawing sedative from a bottle.

following euthanasia such as vocalization or seizures. Alternatively, sedation may be required in order to perform an expedient and effective venipuncture, or provide sufficient restraint for an accurate gunshot or captive bolt stun. Sedation may also make the procedure safer for the operator, handlers, or bystanders.

On the other hand, some individuals feel that sedation may prolong the time it takes for unconsciousness and death, particularly with lethal injection. One argument is that sedation may decrease cardiac output and thus lengthen the time for adequate distribution of the drug. This may result in a period of excitement or continued conscious activity by the patient, which itself can be aversive to onlookers. This may also prolong the time until respiratory and cardiac arrest. These considerations must be evaluated and applied to each case to determine whether or not to sedate an animal prior to euthanasia. Sedation can be applied to any animal undergoing a method of euthanasia that may require mild to moderate chemical restraint. They are more than adequate by themselves for relieving stress and anxiety and many have anal-gesic properties as well. It is only in cases where the technique requires true anesthesia or the pet refuses to relax with a simple sedative, for example, an $\alpha_2$-agonist, will a stronger drug be needed.

For many companion animals, namely dogs, cats, and exotics, pre-euthanasia sedation and anesthesia are helpful on many levels. More and more veterinarians are choosing pre-euthanasia sedation for every dog and cat they euthanize even when the method of euthanasia is acceptable without it. First, animals provided with anesthetic drugs holding analgesic properties are relieved of their physical pain. Families choose euthanasia because their pets are hurting and anesthesia takes that hurt away. It is their time to be as relaxed as possible.

Second, they provide the family some time for physical contact. When an animal is hurting, it often resents being touched and the family misses the connection that only touch can bring. A family may have a pet that never liked to be held and now, when the pet is sleeping, they can do it without resistance.

Lastly, sedation makes the veterinarian's work easier. There is no need to restrain the pet for catheter placement, etc. In the instances where physical methods of euthanasia are used, for example, gunshot, the incidence of improper technique is greatly reduced. Pre-euthanasia sedation minimizes restraint, makes for easier body positioning, and negates the use of more than one person to be present.

## Drugs and routes of administration

Common sedatives administered include $\alpha_2$-agonists, phenothiazines, benzodiazepines, and opiates. Many are often administered in combination for additive effects such as sedation plus analgesia. Dissociative anesthetics such as ketamine and the combination product Telazol® can be used as sedatives, but will lead to complete unconsciousness when given at surgical anesthetic doses. The ones to use for a particular species will be listed within the specific species considerations; see Box 4.2 for a comprehensive list of options.

As mentioned before, many of the pre-euthanasia anesthetic drugs can be combined together for their calming additive effects. The volume administered is based on the individual drug's dosing properties and the weight of the animal being sedated/anesthetized. They can be mixed together in the same syringe and injected intramuscularly (IM) or subcutaneously (SQ). Even those drugs that are labeled for only IM use can be given more gently via the SQ route to the same ultimate effect (Cooney 2011). Sedatives and anesthetics can also be given intravenously(V), keeping in mind that this may cause more stress than it is worth. Some drugs can be given orally in food or squirted in the mouth, as is sometimes needed for fractious dogs and cats (Ramsey and Wetzel 1998). Inhalants are also used to induce unconsciousness in smaller animals. If they are used with large animals, it is usually during a surgical procedure wherein the use of them was not originally intended for pre-euthanasia anesthesia, but rather for surgical anesthesia itself. The goal is to not allow the administration of pre-euthanasia anesthesia to be more stressing than the euthanasia itself.

## Assessing unconsciousness and sedation

How deeply the animal goes into sedation or general anesthesia depends on the type and volume of drugs used.

When the euthanasia method requires unconsciousness, a true anesthetic agent must be administered to guarantee the animal does not respond in any way. Unconsciousness is a state of unawareness or insensibility where the individual is unable to consciously perceive and respond to normal stimuli, including pain.

The unconscious animal is unable to stand and lies recumbent, lacking the ability to right itself to a normal posture. The animal will typically lack normal ocular reflexes including the pupillary light reflex. The lack of normal ocular reflexes indicates disruption of brainstem function and also suggests loss of cerebral cortical function. The animal will lack conscious sensation to pain and thus will not demonstrate a response to painful stimuli such as a needle prick or pinching the ear or extremities. This must be differentiated from simple peripheral reflexes that may still be intact. All of these signs can be quickly assessed during the euthanasia procedure.

Drugs are not required to achieve unconsciousness, but they are used to facilitate it in most instances regarding the euthanasia of client-owned animals. Effective and humane physical methods of inducing unconsciousness, such as penetrating and nonpenetrating captive bolts and electrical stunners often

---

### Box 4.2

#### Signs of unconsciousness
- Recumbency with a lack of a righting reflex
- Absence of a corneal reflex
- Absence of a palpebral reflex
- Loss of spontaneous eye blink
- Absence of eye movement tracking an object
- Fixed and dilated pupils
- Absence of normal rhythmic breathing
- Absence of a pain response

#### Signs of Regaining Consciousness
- Return of coordinated breathing
- Return of corneal or palpebral reflex
- Constricted pupils or return of a pupillary light reflex
- Attempt to raise the head
- Return of a righting reflex
- Return of ocular movement and a blink
- Vocalization
- Response to painful stimulation such as a needle stick

used with livestock and some laboratory animals, render the animal rapidly unconscious. This may then be followed by subsequent death by means of a secondary method such as pithing, administration of KCl, exsanguination, and so on.

If sedation is all that is desired before proceeding with a particular method, the animal will need to be assessed to determine if they are ready for the veterinarian to proceed. Small animals should be calmly lying down with minimal response to stimulation such as auditory, visual, and touch. In the case of large animals, they may remain standing but appear obtunded and uninterested in their surroundings. When little to no response is observed, the veterinarian should feel comfortable proceeding.

## Specific-species considerations

### Dogs and cats

Common injectable sedatives for dogs and cats include the $\alpha_2$-agonists and phenothiazines. They are frequently combined with opiates to enhance sedative and analgesic effects. They can be given SQ, IM, or IV. SQ injections are commonly given between the shoulder blades or under the skin in the lower back or rump area. IM injections are typically given in the epaxial muscles along the back or the lateral thigh. Once administered, their full effects can typically be seen within 5–10 minutes depending on the site of injection and overall health of the pet. Each sedative has common side effects that should be taken into account. For example, dogs and cats are prone to vomiting with $\alpha_2$-agonists, while phenothiazines such as acepromazine may lower cardiac output and mean arterial pressures (Tranquilli and Thurmon 2007). Veterinarians working with dogs and cats should fully review drug pharmacokinetics and pharmacodynamics of their drugs of choice. Note: Common drug doses for dogs and cats can be found in the author's book In-home Pet Euthanasia Techniques (Cooney 2011) or on bottle labels.

Common injectable anesthetics for dogs and cats include propofol and dissociative anesthetics like ketamine, or the combination product Telazol®. Propofol must be administered intravenously typically through an IV catheter, followed shortly after with an injectable euthanasia solution such as pentobarbital. As mentioned before, this is often part of a two-step pre-euthanasia protocol, but may be used alone without a sedative first. Ketamine and Telazol® can be administered SQ, IM, or IV, usually in conjunction with another sedative drug, and should produce reliable anesthesia within 5–10 minutes. Ketamine and Telazol® are not labeled for SQ injection, but work effectively in dogs and cats via this route for the purpose of pre-euthanasia anesthesia (Figure 4.2; Cooney 2011). Both have the potential to sting when administered SQ or IM, so clients should be warned their pet may react briefly. Sedatives and anesthetics should be administered slowly with small gauge needles to minimize pain on injection.

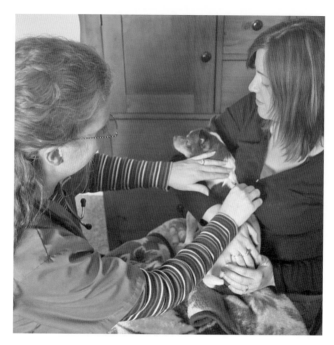

**Figure 4.2** Subcutaneous injection of an anesthetic in a small dog.

Common inhalant anesthetics, like isoflurane, halothane, and sevoflurane, can be administered to small dogs, cats, and newborn puppies and kittens. They may be placed within chambers or made to breathe in using facemasks. They should be fully assessed for unconsciousness before proceeding.

Running fingers and hands gently along the pet's body can easily assess the depth of sedation and anesthesia. Other methods include toe pinching, tickling in between the toe pads, or touching the caudal thigh to check for tail tucking. Dogs and cats generally keep their eyes open during this time even though they remain unresponsive. They may blink when the medial canthus is touched during sedation, but they should remain unresponsive in deep anesthesia. Some will urinate and defecate in direct response to the level of relaxation and the drugs used.

## Exotics

### Ferrets

If the ferret is too active and alert for gas anesthesia, an injectable sedative should be used. Generally, 0.1 cc dexmedetomidine and 0.1 cc butorphanol mixed in the same syringe with a 25-gauge needle given IM works very rapidly and usually does not sting. For an IM injection, the ferret can be scruffed by gently gripping a fold of skin over the dorsal neck, which will normally cause the ferret to relax like a cat. The most accessible muscle to use is the thigh muscle. The leg can be firmly held while the needle is inserted. This must be done quickly in order to minimize stress for the ferret and prevent injury to the handler, as the ferret may try to bite. The aforementioned drug combination may be used SQ though it can take up to 20-25 minutes to take affect. SQ injections may be easier to administer, although the volume of drug needs to be much higher for dexmedetomidine to take effect. Whatever route is chosen, being quick with the injection and confident with the handling of the ferret is important.

Other options of drugs are xylazine (20 mg/mL)/ketamine (100 mg/mL) 1:5 by volume mix given IM at a dose of 0.13 mL per1100-g ferret (Rhoades 2002), or Telazol® 0.15 mL combined with acepromazine 0.05 mL given SQ. These drugs may sting when given IM or SQ causing a reaction in front of the owner. The owner should be forewarned of this reaction but these combinations of drugs are generally more rapid to affect given SQ than the dexmedetomidine, usually reaching full sedation within 5-10 minutes.

## Rabbits

Rabbits tend to take longer than other exotics to relax into unconsciousness or heavy sedation. Sedative drugs can be administered IM using the lumbar mus-cles or quadriceps muscles, or SQ within the shoulder blade region. Injectable sedation drugs include dexmedetomidine and butorphanol at 0.1 mL of each given IM. This produces sedation within 5-10 minutes. Telazol® 0.3-0.4 mL combined with acepromazine 0.1 mL given SQ produces full anesthesia within 5 minutes. Once the rabbit is fully unconscious, the barbiturate solution can be administered IV, IP, IC, or intraorgan.

## Guinea pigs, chinchillas, rats, hamsters, gerbils, mice, and sugar gliders

In many cases, a cotton ball soaked with a liquid gas anesthestic placed in a chamber or anesthesia mask is the quickest, fastest, and least stressful way to anesthetize some of these very small animals. This can then be followed up with an IP or intraorgan injection of euthanasia fluid if necessary.

If liquid gas anesthesia is not available, a SQ injection of a sedative or anesthetic can be given. Keep in mind the handling of the small mammals can be stressful and challenging, especially in the sugar gliders and mice. This sedation would then be followed with an IP or intrahepatic injection of the euthanasia drug.

## Reptiles

If the reptile is very cold, due to its slow metabolism, it should be warmed prior to sedation/anesthesia in order to speed up the rate of uptake of the drug. This can be done using a heating pad on the lowest setting and wrapping the animal with the heating pad and a towel to secure it. Warming can also be accomplished with the use of warm wet towels in baggies wrapped around the animal. A snake can be placed in a plastic tube and have a warm towel or heating pad placed around the tube to warm it. It may take up to 20-45 minutes to warm the animal to at least room temperature, depending on how debilitated it is. During this time, it is helpful to place a doplar unit in order to locate the heartbeat prior to sedation. Warming the reptile to room temperature will help the sedation drugs take effect within 15-20 minutes

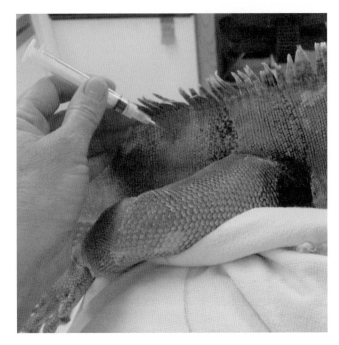

**Figure 4.3** Intramuscular (IM) injection into the lumbar muscle of an iguana.

(Mader 1996). A reminder here that reptiles do not accept inhalant agents easily and will not achieve consistent sedation or anesthesia from them.

Anesthesia prior to euthanizing may be warranted for larger, more difficult to handle, or potentially dangerous reptiles, and for IC injections. These drugs include Telazol® at 25 mg/kg IM and ketamine at 100-200 mg/kg IM. Anesthesia for lizards can be accomplished with an IM injection into the lumbar muscle group, the thigh muscle group, or the front leg into the biceps muscle group (Figures 4.3-4.5). Given reptile's slow metabolism and ability to hold their breath for long periods of time, euthanasia or sedation using inhalant anesthesia is generally not recommended.

For snakes, an IM injection can be given into the epaxial muscles along the spine (Figure 4.6). Chelonians can be given sedative injections into the front limb using the biceps or triceps muscles (Figures 4.7).

### Birds

For birds weighing over 750 g, they can be relaxed using IM injections of ketamine or Telazol® or combination of drugs such as dexmedetomidine combined with nalbuphine, butorphanol, or ketamine. Any of these drugs will give good sedation, which can then be followed by an injection of a barbiturate given either IV, IC, or directly into the liver; see Table 4.1 for doses.

*Medetomidine*: Dose varies between species of birds, 200-300 mg/kg, with ketamine at dose of 5-10 mg/kg IM or IV.
*Ketamine*: Dose range depends on species of birds, between 10 and 75 mg/kg IM or IV, with diazepam at 0.5-2.5 mg/kg.

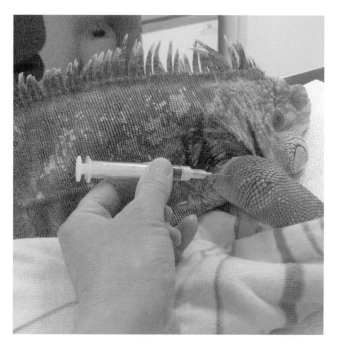

**Figure 4.4** Biceps muscle injection.

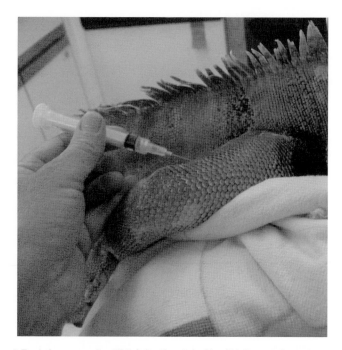

**Figure 4.5** Intramuscular (IM) injection into the thigh muscle group.

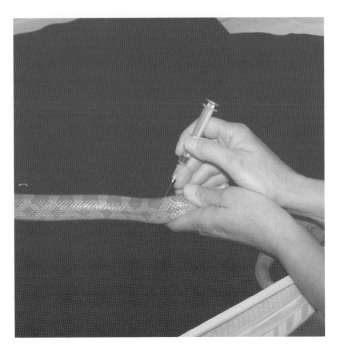

**Figure 4.6** Intramuscular (IM) injection into the epaxial muscle.

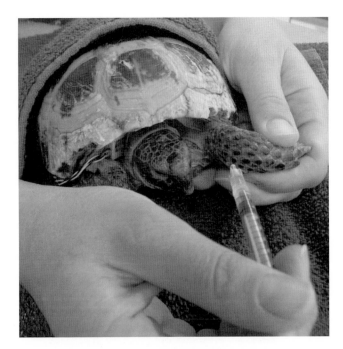

**Figure 4.7** Intramuscular (IM) injection into the muscle of the forelimb of a tortoise.

**Table 4.1** Reasons for and against pre-euthanasia sedation or anesthesia in domestic animals (generalized).

| Method of anesthesia/euthanasia | Ferrets | Rabbits | Rodents/guinea pigs | Reptiles | Amphibian | Avian <150 g | Avian >150 g | Fish |
|---|---|---|---|---|---|---|---|---|
| Inhalant anesthesia: $CO_2$ | Flow rate: 20% vol/min | Flow rate: 20% vol/min | | | | | | To effect |
| Inhalant anesthesia: soaked cotton ball | To effect | To effect | To effect | Not effective | To effect | To effect | For sedation | |
| Butorphenol/dexmetomadine | 0.1 mL/0.1 mL, IM | 0.3-0.4 mL of each, IM | 0.1-0.2 mL of each, IM | | | | | |
| Ketamine/dexmetomadine | | | | | | | 5-10 mg/kg, 200-300 mg/kg, IV, IM | |
| Telazol | | | | 25 mg/kg, IM | | 0.11 mL/kg, IM | 0.11 mL/kg, IM | |
| Telazol/acepromazine | 0.15 mL/0.05 mL, SQ | 0.3-0.4 mL/0.1 mL, SQ | | | | | | |
| Ketamine | | | | 100-200 mg/kg, IM | | 0.2-0.4 mL (20-40 mg), IM | 0.3 mg/g, IM | |
| Xylazine (20 mg/mL)/ketamine (100 mg/mL), 1:5 mixture | 0.13 mL/100 g ferret, IM | 0.5 mL/10#, IM | 0.5 mL/10#, IM | | | 0.11 mL/kg, IM | 0.11 mL/kg, IM | |
| Barbiturate overdose (3× anesthetic dose) | 120 mg/kg, IV, IP | 100 mg/kg, IV; 150 mg/kg, IP | 150 mg/kg, IV, IP | 100 or >100 mg/kg, IV, IP | 100 or >100 mg/kg, IV, ICo | 0.22 mL/kg, IV, IP | 0.22 mL/kg, IV, IP | 100 mg/kg, IP, IV |

(continued)

**Table 4.1** (continued)

| Method of anesthesia/euthanasia | Ferrets | Rabbits | Rodents/guinea pigs | Reptiles | Amphibian | Avian <150 g | Avian >150 g | Fish |
|---|---|---|---|---|---|---|---|---|
| Commercial euthanasia solution | 0.22 mL/kg, IV, IP | 0.22 mL/kg, IV, IP | 0.22 mL/kg, IV, IP | 200 mg/kg, IV, IP | 0.22 mL/kg, IV, ICo, IC | 0.22 mL/kg, IV, IP | 0.22 mL/kg, IV, IP | 100 mg/kg, IP, IV |
| Benzocain hydrochloride, 250 mg/l water bath | | | | | Soak to effect | | | |
| Tricane methane sulphonate MS-222®, 3 g/L | | | | | Soak to effect | | | |
| KCl, IV or IC, in anesthetized animal | | | | 75-150 mg/kg KCl | | | | 75-150 mg/kg KCl |
| Unacceptable methods<br>Stunning in an awake animal<br>Electrocution in an awake animal<br>Drowning in an awake animal<br>Freezing in an awake animal<br>Kitchen microwave oven<br>Cervical dislocation, decapitation >500 g animal<br>Exsanguination in an awake animal<br>$CO_2$ using dry ice: need $CO_2$ chamber | | | | | | | | |

IM, intramuscular; IP, intraperitoneal; IV, intravenous; SQ, subcutaneous; ICo, Intracoelomic.

Length of time for induction of sedation and anesthesia varies with route of administration, drugs used, and the species being sedated. In some birds, the injectable sedatives will be enough to cause death, especially if the doses are at the high end of the ranges and the bird's condition is poor. Once adequate unconsciousness has been achieved, the barbiturate drug can then be administered. This can be given IV or intrahepatic.

For sedation drugs to be administered, IM or Intracoelomic (ICo) injections are quite easy for the clinician less skilled in IV administration. IM injections are given into the pectoral muscles that cover the keel bone. These muscles are quite large unless the bird is severely debilitated and in these cases the thigh muscles can be used. The bird is wrapped in a towel and the pectoral muscles can be located by palpating the keel bone and the muscles are on either side. Be sure to locate the soft crop area proximal to the point of the keel bone and be sure not to inject in that region for the absorption of drug will be much slower. Once the pectoral muscle is located, a 0.5-1-in., 27-22-gauge needle (depending on the size of the bird) is inserted perpendicular to the skin. The needle can be inserted to the hub, if it is inserted too deep, bone will be encountered and the needle should be withdrawn slightly before injecting. For the larger birds that are much more stressed when picked up, the pectoral muscles can be located with the bird standing, taking care that the wings are firmly controlled with a large towel. The clinician can follow the keel bone down to the largest portion of the pectoral muscles and inject the drug (Figure 4.8). This is done by using a blind insertion since the pectoral

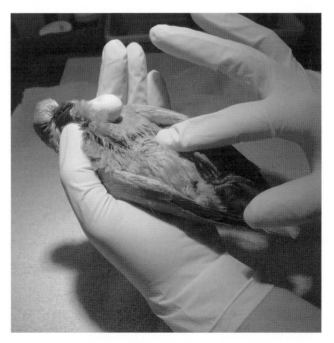

**Figure 4.8** The pectoral muscles can be located on either side of the keel bone.

muscles are going to be ventral. This is a much less stressful way to handle these large birds and much safer for personnel.

## Horses

A local anesthetic or mild sedative may facilitate the placing of an IV catheter or allow for easier direct venipuncture. Sedation may be used to lower the horse's head for improved gunshot and captive bolt positioning. It can be useful for restraint during euthanasia, but veterinarians must acknowledge that there may be a depressant effect from sedation on the circulatory system, which may increase the time required for the animal to lose consciousness. It is good to warn the client that there may also be an increased amount of muscular activity and agonal gasping when euthanizing a sedated horse. Sedation should still be used for excited or untrained horses or for horses in severe pain as from colic.

Sedation of horses to facilitate euthanasia has been an area of controversy among equine veterinarians. Sedation may make the horse more easily managed, but does have certain disadvantages. Sedation may not be safely or practically administered to wild or untrained horses in many cases. The increased cost incurred by some sedatives may be a significant disadvantage for some owners. Also, many believe that euthanasia is delayed by the cardiovascular depression of most sedatives.

If sedation is chosen, the $\alpha_2$-agonist group of sedatives is most commonly employed. Xylazine is very inexpensive and provides adequate sedation for most equids. The dose may range from 0.4 mg/kg to 1.1 mg/kg IV. In many cases, the doses in the lower end of the spectrum will effect adequate sedation without the ataxia often seen with the higher doses. Detomidine is a much more profound sedative, but is significantly more expensive. Label dosage is 20 or 40 mcg/kg IV. As with xylazine, the higher doses may produce ataxia. Both of these drugs may be given IM at the upper dosage if IV administration is impossible (Figure 4.9). With IM administration, sedation is more variable and the onset will be delayed. Other less commonly used sedatives such as acepromazine or romifidine may be used at labeled dosages. Sedation in donkeys and mules does not last as long as horses, so larger doses may be required.

## Livestock

Pre-euthanasia sedation is typically used in livestock in order to aid in restraint and improve safety for the veterinarian, owner, and other bystanders. In some cases of pet livestock, the owner may request sedation prior to euthanasia. In many cases, only mild sedation is needed to allow for successful venipuncture, catheter placement, or accurate gunshot or stunning. With more excitable animals, deep sedation may be required to ensure that the animal remains recumbent for the procedure in order to provide adequate restraint and safety.

$\alpha_2$-agonists, such as xylazine, are probably the most common sedative used for livestock. Xylazine provides potent sedation along with analgesia at very low doses in ruminants and camelids. Acepromazine can also be used but

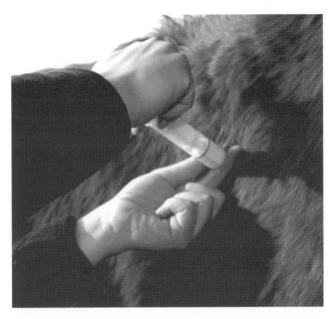

**Figure 4.9** Intramuscular injection of a sedative in the neck of a horse.

will not provide additional analgesia and will result in vasodilation and hypotension. Benzodiazepines such as diazepam or midazolam are also effective sedatives in ruminant and camelid species. Opioids such as morphine or butorphanol will also provide sedation and analgesia. Of all the livestock species, sedation of swine is probably the most unpredictable and may require high doses to obtain the desired effect. Combinations of sedatives are often used to provide more consistent and effective sedation and analgesia, particularly in pigs.

In rare circumstances, general anesthesia may be preferred to sedation prior to euthanasia of livestock. In some cases, this is simply because the animal is undergoing general anesthesia for a surgical procedure. Another example is euthanasia of pigs where the restraint needed to successfully perform venipuncture, insert an IV catheter, or perform an IC injection cannot be obtained with sedation alone. Injectable anesthetics such as ketamine and Telazol are effective and commonly used in ruminants, camelids, and swine. Inhalation anesthetics such as isoflurane are effective in livestock as well.

As in horses, the cardiovascular and respiratory depressant effects of sedatives or general anesthesia have the potential to prolong the duration of subsequent euthanasia when using injection of pentobarbital-containing solutions. Clients should be forewarned of this when using these drugs.

## Cattle
In many instances, it may not be possible to safely restrain the animal simply with a halter or lariat or when an appropriate chute with a side opening is not available. In these cases, immobilization with sedation is required. A variety of drugs and drug combinations can be used for this, some of which are listed in Table 4.2. Xylazine is a common inexpensive sedative analgesic

**Table 4.2** Some suggested drugs and drug combinations for providing standing or recumbent sedation prior to euthanasia in cattle.

| Drug or drug combination | Dosage and route | Comments |
| --- | --- | --- |
| Xylazine | 0.01–0.05 mg/kg, IV<br>0.01–0.1 mg/kg, IM | Standing sedation. Dosage dependent on the excitability of the animal. |
| | 0.1–0.2 mg/kg, IV or IM | Results in recumbency in most cattle. Higher doses can be used in anxious animals to assure recumbency prior to euthanasia. |
| Detomidine | 0.002–0.02 mg/kg, IV or IM | Standing sedation. Dosage dependent on the excitability of the animal. |
| Acepromazine | 0.05–0.1 mg/kg, IV or IM | Will provide sedation but no analgesia. Marked hypotension may prolong euthanasia by injectable barbiturates. |
| Standing Ket-Stun<br>  Butorphanol<br>  Xylazine<br>  Ketamine | Combine for SQ or IM injection (1:2:4 ratio)<br>0.01–0.025 mg/kg<br>0.02–0.05 mg/kg<br>0.04–0.10 mg/kg | Provides effective standing sedation and chemical restraint for most cattle. Anxious cattle may need a higher dose. Increasing xylazine increases the likelihood of recumbency. |
| Recumbent Ket-Stun<br>  Butorphanol<br>  Xylazine<br>  Ketamine | Combine for SQ or IM injection.<br>0.025 mg/kg<br>0.05 mg/kg<br>0.1 mg/kg | Routinely provides sedation and recumbency in most cattle. Onset in 3–10 min. |
| Xylazine-ketamine combination | Xylazine 0.05 mg/kg, IV<br>Ketamine 4.5 mg/kg, IV | Produces rapid anesthesia that will last for 15–20 min. |
| TKX-ruminant<br>  Telazol<br>  Ketamine<br>  Xylazine | Reconstitute a 500 mg vial of Telazol with 250 mg (2.5 mL) ketamine and 100 mg (1 mL) xylazine. Administer at 1–1.5 mL/110 kg, IM | Recumbency in 5–10 min. The low volume makes this combination ideal for immobilizing intractable ruminants. It may be administered by syringe, with a pole syringe, or dart gun if needed. Relatively expensive. |

IM, intramuscular; IV, intravenous; SQ, subcutaneous.

used in livestock. It provides reliable sedation and will result in predictable recumbency with relatively low doses and low cost. Detomidine is another $\alpha_2$-adrenergic agonist sedative that could be used for sedation and restraint. However, detomidine is more expensive and results in greater cardiorespiratory depression that may result in prolonged response to lethal injection with barbiturates. Acepromazine is also an effective sedative in cattle but does not provide any significant analgesia. In addition, the hypotension resulting from inhibition of catecholamine-mediated vascular tone may result in prolonged response to lethal injection. Combinations of xylazine, butorphanol, and ketamine (Ket-Stun protocols) and Telazol®, ketamine, and xylazine (TKX protocols) can be used for reliable standing and recumbent restraint in cattle. Such combinations can provide profound sedation and analgesia.

In some instances, the animal may not be safely approached in order to administer sedation directly. Examples would be some range beef cattle, rodeo cattle, and bison. In these situations, the animals are generally very excitable and may override simple sedation with just xylazine. A pole syringe or dart gun may be necessary for safe sedation in these animals. The drug chambers for pole syringes and dart guns are often limited in the volume that can be administered. The low volume required for TKX protocols is advantageous for sedation and recumbency in these excitable and potentially dangerous animals. Otherwise, euthanasia by gunshot at longer range with a hunting rifle might be most appropriate.

### Sheep and goats

Sedation is rarely necessary in euthanasia of sheep and goats except in the most excitable animals such as wild sheep and goats. Similar sedatives as used in cattle can be used in sheep and goats with similar considerations. A list of several options for small ruminants is listed in Table 4.3.

### Pigs

Consistent sedation in pigs can be challenging. Pigs tend to have erratic responses to most livestock sedatives. However, since the pig is going to be euthanized, high doses can be used without harm. Alternatively, combinations of sedatives and anesthetics seem to provide more consistent results. Common injectable sedatives and anesthetics used in swine are presented in Table 4.4. IV injection can be challenging in pigs. Common sites include the ear vein, the anterior vena cava, brachiocephalic vein, jugular vein, coccygeal vein, cephalic vein, or lateral saphenous vein.

Vietnamese pot-bellied pigs or other pet pigs present additional challenges for euthanasia. They tend to resist physical restraint and they also tend to have poorly visible ear veins for venipuncture. In addition, the family may want to be present and will expect the procedure to be performed with minimal distress for their pet. A very acceptable approach to euthanasia of pet pigs is to first induce general anesthesia followed by venipuncture or IC injection of pentobarbital euthanasia solution or a saturated KCl solution. General anesthesia may be induced using various drug combinations administered IM behind the

**Table 4.3** Some suggested drugs and drug combinations for providing standing or recumbent sedation prior to euthanasia in small ruminants.

| Drug or drug combination | Dosage and route | Comments |
|---|---|---|
| Xylazine | 0.01–0.05 mg/kg, IV<br>0.01–0.1 mg/kg, IM | Standing sedation. Dosage dependent on the excitability of the animal. |
| | 0.1–0.2 mg/kg, IV or IM | Results in recumbency in most cattle. Higher doses can be used in anxious animals to assure recumbency prior to euthanasia. |
| Detomidine | 0.002–0.02 mg/kg, IV or IM | Standing sedation. Dosage dependent on the excitability of the animal. |
| Acepromazine | 0.05–0.1 mg/kg, IV or IM | Will provide sedation but no analgesia. Marked hypotension may prolong euthanasia by injectable barbiturates. |
| Diazepam or midazolam | 0.2–0.4 mg/kg, IV<br>0.3–0.5 mg/kg, IM | Provides moderate sedation in most sheep and goats. |
| Sheep Ket-Stun<br>  Butorphanol<br>  Xylazine<br>  Ketamine | Combine for SQ or IM injection<br>0.025 mg/kg<br>0.05 mg/kg<br>1.0 mg/kg | Provides conscious sedation while significantly limiting movement in the animal. The animal will often become recumbent. |
| Small-ruminant cocktail | Combine ketamine (100 mg/mL), xylazine (100 mg/mL), and butorphanol (10 mg/mL) at a 10:1:1 ratio. Administer at 1 mL/80–100 lb BW IM. If giving IV, start with 2/3 dose. | Provides recumbency and good anesthesia in 5–10 min in most sheep and goats. |
| Xylazine-ketamine combination | Xylazine 0.05 mg/kg, IV<br>Ketamine 4.5 mg/kg, IV | Produces rapid anesthesia that will last for 15–20 min. |
| TKX-ruminant<br>  Telazol<br>  Ketamine<br>  Xylazine | Reconstitute a 500 mg vial of Telazol with 250 mg (2.5 mL) ketamine and 100 mg (1 mL) xylazine. Administer at 1–1.5 mL/110 kg, IM | Recumbency in 5–10 min. The low volume makes this combination ideal for immobilizing intractable ruminants. It may be administered by syringe, with a pole syringe, or dart gun if needed. Relatively expensive. |

IM, intramuscular; IV, intravenous; SQ, subcutaneous; BW, body weight.

**Table 4.4** Some suggested drugs and drug combinations for providing sedation or anesthesia prior to euthanasia in pigs.

| Drug or drug combination | Dosage and route | Comments |
|---|---|---|
| Acepromazine | 0.5-5 mg/kg, IM | Will provide sedation but no analgesia. Marked hypotension may prolong euthanasia by injectable barbiturates. |
| Diazepam or midazolam | 0.2-1 mg/kg, IM | Provides moderate sedation and muscle relaxation in most pigs. |
| Xylazine | 0.5-3.0 mg/kg, IM | Sedation, but unreliable when used alone. |
| Diazepam/midazolam plus butorphenol/morphine | 0.2-0.5 mg/kg, IM 0.2-0.5 mg/kg, IM | This IM combination will generally provide smooth sedation. Good prior to masking with isoflurane. |
| Detomidine Midazolam Butorphanol | 20-60 $\mu$g/kg, IM 0.3 mg/kg, IM 0.3 mg/kg, IM | This drug combination provides deep sedation. |
| Swine Telazol cocktail | Suspend a 500 mg vial of Telazol with 2.5 mL ketamine (100 mg/mL) and 2.5 mL xylazine (100 mg/mL). Administer at 1 mL/35 kg, IM | Smooth anesthesia. Apnea may occur. |
| Midazolam Telazol | 5 mg/kg, IM 4 mg/kg, IM | This combination induces anesthesia in most pigs. |

IM, intramuscular.

ear in the neck. Alternatively, many pigs accept being masked with isoflurane. This may be done with or without sedation administered by IM injection. Intramuscular or subcutaneous injections are most commonly administered in the neck just caudal to the ear in pigs.

## Llamas and alpacas

Because the jugular vein can be difficult to hit in llamas and alpacas, and because the carotid artery is positioned very close to the jugular vein, initial sedation is often given by the SQ or IM route. Intracarotid injection of the sedatives will result in rapid excitement and possibly seizure activity. If giving

**Table 4.5** Some suggested drugs and drug combinations for providing standing or recumbent sedation prior to euthanasia in llamas and alpacas.

| Drug or drug combination | Dosage and route | Comments |
|---|---|---|
| Xylazine | 0.05–0.1 mg/kg, IV 0.1–0.4 mg/kg, IM or SQ | Standing or recumbent sedation. Dosage dependent on the excitability of the animal. |
| Butorphanol | 0.05–0.2 mg/kg, IV or IM or SQ | Produces sedation, and at the higher doses may produce recumbency. |
| Diazepam or midazolam | 0.2–0.4 mg/kg, IV 0.3–0.5 mg/kg, IM or SQ | Provides moderate sedation in most sheep and goats. |
| Camelid Ket-Stun Butorphanol Xylazine Ketamine | Combine for SQ or IM injection (1:2:4 ratio) 0.05–0.1 mg/kg 0.1–0.2 mg/kg 0.2–0.4 mg/kg | Provides conscious sedation. Animal may stay standing or become recumbent. |
| Small-ruminant cocktail | Combine ketamine (100 mg/mL), xylazine (100 mg/mL), and butorphanol (10 mg/mL) at a 10:1:1 ratio. Administer at 1 mL/50 lb BW in llamas and 1 mL/40 lb BW in alpacas IM. If giving IV, start with 2/3 dose. | This same mixture that is used in small ruminants is very effective in llamas and alpacas as well, just at a higher dosage. Provides recumbency and good anesthesia in 5–10 min in most llamas and alpacas. |
| Diazepam-ketamine combination | Diazepam 0.1–0.2 mg/kg, IV Ketamine 3 mg/kg, IV | Produces rapid anesthesia that will last for 15–20 min. |

IM, intramuscular; IV, intravenous; SQ, subcutaneous; BW, body weight.

the initial sedation intravenously by the jugular vein, it is recommended to initially give small portions of the dose slowly to check for an adverse response before the bulk of the drug is administered. Sites for IM injections are the triceps and the semimembranosus and semitendinosus muscles. SQ injections can be given in the neck, just in front of the shoulder, over the triceps, or over the caudal thigh (see Table 4.5).

# Chapter 5
# Euthanasia Techniques

**V**eterinarians and staff are encouraged to have standard protocols in place that clearly outline the methods used and reasons for them. All methods of euthanasia have the potential to be poorly performed if personnel have not been properly trained. Those performing euthanasia should be monitored for proficiency and emotional fortitude and encouraged to gain further skills through advanced training for the benefit of the animal and client. As previously mentioned in Chapter 3, understanding animal behavior and restraint techniques will help facilitate a smoother procedure.

The following techniques are segmented into euthanasia by inhalant agents, noninhalant pharmaceutical agents, and physical methods. Because owners are commonly present during euthanasia (Adams et al. 2000), the manner of death in front of onlookers should be taken into consideration. With any of these techniques, those administering the technique should take their time and be consistent. If one technique proves challenging, another can be attempted to ensure that a proper euthanasia takes place, both for animal and client's sake. The techniques are described in such a way as to demonstrate the ideal manner of protocol. Because it is impossible to guarantee that every attempt will be perfect, there is a section on technical challenges following each method. This will provide insight on how best to move forward with euthanasia in difficult situations.

## How death is achieved

The reason that these techniques are listed as methods of euthanasia is that they all lead to cardiac death in the patient. The manner in which this happens is unique to each technique, even if the differences appear rather subtle. Euthanasia is achieved through (1) direct depression of neurons necessary for life, (2) hypoxia, and (3) physical disruption of brain activity. To be considered euthanasia, as mentioned before, the animal must be allowed to die in the most pain-free and stress-free manner possible. Circumstances will dictate how ideally the euthanasia method may be carried out.

*Veterinary Euthanasia Techniques: A Practical Guide*, First Edition. Kathleen A. Cooney, Jolynn R. Chappell, Robert J. Callan and Bruce A. Connally.
© 2012 John Wiley & Sons, Inc. Published 2012 by John Wiley & Sons, Inc.

## Direct depression of neurons necessary for life

- *Injectable agents*: barbiturates, T-61®, Tributame®
- *Immersion/topical agents*: benzocaine hydrochloride (HCl), tricaine methanesulfonate (MS-222)
- *Anesthetic agents*: both inhalants (e.g., halothane) and injectable agents (e.g., propofol)

Mechanism of action: Euthanasia by these agents is basically an overdose of an anesthetic. The animal will first become unconscious due to suppression of the cerebral cortex. A state of general anesthesia and unconsciousness can be assessed by the lack of a corneal and palpebral reflex. The progression from consciousness, to recumbency, to unconsciousness is generally smooth and progressive with current euthanasia solutions when administered appropriately. Early stages of anesthesia may lead to an excitatory phase producing dysphoria, mild to severe muscle movement, and vocalization. Respiration rate is initially decreased and progresses to a more erratic respiratory pattern along with an identifiable heartbeat. As death ensues, a few final deep respiratory gasps may be observed in many species. Generally, respiratory arrest is observed prior to cardiac arrest when euthanasia is performed with these agents. Because of the potential for recovery, care must be taken to ensure that death has occurred prior to disposing of animal remains.

## Hypoxia

- *Inert gases*: carbon dioxide ($CO_2$), nitrogen (N), argon (Ar), and carbon monoxide (CO)
- *Physical methods*: exsanguination, decapitation, and potassium chloride (KCl)

Mechanisms of action: Inhalant gases such as $CO_2$, N, and Ar displace oxygen within the chamber or mask leading to direct hypoxia. CO works differently by binding to red blood cells to form carboxyhemoglobin, thus blocking oxygen binding. Exsanguination and decapitation halt blood flow to the brain and cardiac muscle leading to death. KCl causes direct cardiac arrest, ultimately ceasing blood flow.

## Physical disruption of brain activity

- *Concussive stunning*: blow to the head and electrical stunning
- *Direct destruction*: gunshot, captive bolt, pithing, and freezing
- *Depolarization of neurons*: electrocution (not included in this book)

Mechanisms of action: Direct destruction of brain tissue leads to immediate death as long as the medullary centers within the brainstem are also destroyed. Concussive stunning renders the animal unconscious when done properly. These methods must be followed by a secondary method of euthanasia such as exsanguination. Depolarization of neurons through electrocution is a conditionally acceptable method in some animals, but will not be discussed here due to its limited use in general practice.

## Choosing an appropriate method

The method of euthanasia chosen by the veterinarian will depend on many things such as the following:

- Comfort with the technique
- Supplies
- The presence of onlookers
- The type and amount of euthanasia drug available
- The signalment and physical condition of the animal
- The need for a postmortem examination

### Comfort with the technique

When a veterinarian has experience with a particular technique, they know what to expect and how to handle the situation if something unexpected happens. All veterinarians should know at least two other methods in case circumstances indicate another technique is needed. Experience is gained with every euthanasia, but if something unexpected occurs, the attending veterinarian and staff should be educated on how to proceed in the animal's best interest. Each technique has pros and cons depending on these factors. The veterinarian, along with some client input if acceptable, must decide which technique to use. Only by attempting one technique will the veterinarian come to understand if another technique must be used instead, given the circumstances.

### Supplies

As supplies are prepared, things should be included for a standard euthanasia procedure as well as emergency equipment. For injectable methods, various needle sizes, syringes, catheters, cleaning gauze, etc., need to be accessible at all times. For physical methods, the equipment must be cleaned and ready for use. Veterinarians are encouraged to keep ample supply of all materials within the euthanasia room, in mobile-supply bags, etc. Depending on the animal being aided, this includes keeping enough inhalants, euthanasia solution, or bullets in stock to avoid the inability to carry out the procedure.

### The presence of onlookers

Veterinarians know that as long as an animal is sedated or unconscious, most methods of euthanasia are humane. As long as death is as stress free and pain free as possible, and timely, any of the approved methods are acceptable.

However, when family members and clients are watching, the least aversive technique available should be chosen for that particular species. As long as it is explained to the client how the procedure will take place and the approximate time frame involved, most clients will be acceptable to the method chosen. Keeping communication open and answering any questions they may have will help to decrease their stress. Sometimes, the clinician needs to prompt these questions due to the client's state of mind, as they may not think of things to ask. When a slower method is chosen, such as an intraperitoneal (IP) injection, onlookers should be prepared that death may take a few minutes. When venous access is impossible, due to poor pressures, overlying masses, small size of the animal, etc., intracardiac (IC) injections are commonly done. In the case of large animals, gunshot is often the most practical method, but the reaction of onlookers must be considered. Clients/family members typically handle the technique very well when they understand why it is done and that their animal remains comfortable throughout. Once again, education is important to lessen fears of the unknown.

## The type and amount of euthanasia solution available

Domesticated animal euthanasia is most commonly carried out using barbiturates or barbiturate-combination drugs. It is considered the most acceptable method, except for those intended for food use. All euthanasia solution labels should be fully understood before use. With proper pre-euthanasia anesthesia, barbiturates are approved for all injectable methods: IV, IC, IP, and intraorgan injections. If pre-euthanasia sedation or anesthesia is not available, barbiturate-combination drugs, such as those with phenytoin sodium, are not approved for IP use. The additive may cause cardiac arrest before the pet goes unconscious, thus leading to distress. KCl must be given IV or IC under complete anesthesia. Factors such as these should be understood before euthanasia is performed in any situation.

The amount of solution available is also important. Euthanasia should never be attempted without adequate amounts of solution ready for use. Each drug has a standard dosing protocol for each technique that needs to be strictly followed to achieve proper euthanasia parameters. For example, IP injections using pentobarbital require a dosing of 3 mL per 10 lb of body mass versus the more standard IV amount of 1 mL per 10 lb (Fakkema 2008). If improper levels of solution are administered, the animal may recover, causing distress to the animal, family, veterinary staff, and aftercare facility operators. Instances such as these lead to distrust by the public and negatively impact the general perception of euthanasia by those considering it for their own animal.

If only a small amount of euthanasia solution is available, a technique should be chosen that requires the smallest volume possible, such as an IV injection. IC injections can be tricky, especially if it is difficult to locate the heart and the solution ends up in the lungs or pleural space. If there is not enough solution, the veterinarian will be unable to complete the euthanasia.

## The signalment and physical condition of the animal

The signalment and physical condition of the animal being euthanized should always be a factor when choosing the euthanasia technique. Weight, size, disease, species, and even breed, all contribute to how well a particular technique can be expected to work. Following are a few examples of differences that veterinarians will encounter:

- *Weight*: Obesity makes veins harder to see and feel, makes the chest wall thicker, creates large amounts of intra-abdominal fat, and may lead to increased dyspnea during sedation/anesthesia. If the patient is an overweight cat, choosing an IV injection rather than an intrarenal injection might be advantageous because finding and isolating a kidney can be difficult. The sheer weight of some large animals can make working with them safely almost impossible and methods must be modified to protect staff and the animal itself.
- *Size*: When one is considering the length of veins, short-legged dog breeds are harder to euthanize than long-legged breeds. Small birds will have smaller, more delicate veins than larger birds, and so on. For obvious reasons, IC injections are rarely, if ever, attempted on large animals. Size will also impact whether an animal can fit into an inhalation chamber, be euthanized with a .22 pistol versus a larger gun, etc.
- *Age*: Age can affect technique. Young neonates are difficult, if not impossible, to gain IV access on. An inhalant agent or IP injection of a barbiturate might be more commonly used in young animals. Young livestock may be easier to euthanize with a physical method due to their softer craniums. An older animal may be naturally weaker and have an underlying disease of some sort, forcing the veterinarian to tailor methods accordingly.
- *Disease*: The presence of illness, be it heart disease, cancer, renal failure, etc., can affect blood pressure, circulation, perfusion, and drug uptake. If the animal has extremely low blood pressure, the veins might be inaccessible. If the heart wall is thickened, or is surrounded by a tumor or a hemopericardium, an IC injection is more difficult. When peripheral edema is present, veins may be virtually impossible to find making it necessary to abandon an IV injection altogether. If a small animal has ascites or hemoabdomen, an IP injection will be diluted into the abdominal fluid likely leading to a prolonged time of death, and so on.

Another factor to consider is how well the animal will tolerate pre-euthanasia sedation or anesthesia. If the animal in question is having a hard time breathing, a technique should be chosen that allows for rapid euthanasia before the dyspnea worsens. It is hard to watch an animal struggle to breathe while waiting for an IP injection to stop the heart. The same is true for seizuring animals or any other crisis situation that may present. For this reason, drugs and their associated side effects should be well understood before using them.

- *Species*: In most cases, dogs and cats are euthanized easily by IV, IC, or intra-abdominal injections. In general, intrarenal injections are easier to perform in cats due to their freely movable left kidney resting outside the retroperitoneal space (Cooney 2011). Swine can be difficult to control negating the need for pre-euthanasia sedation or anesthesia. Inhalant gases are not recommended for use with reptiles and amphibians, and so on.
- *Breeds*: Different breeds vary in their physical and physiological attributes; leg length, head shape, hair coat, predisposition to disease, etc., all play a role in determining which euthanasia technique is the most appropriate. For example, brachycephalic dogs and cats have a tendency to become dyspneic under pre-euthanasia sedation/anesthesia and also may overheat when outdoors or lying in front of the fire. It can be nearly impossible for an inexperienced veterinarian to locate the jugular vein on a sheep due to its thick wool, and if clippers are not present, a physical method might be required, and so on.

## The need for a postmortem examination

It is important to know whether or not an animal will be studied following euthanasia. If so, techniques should be chosen that minimize organ and tissue damage. When using a euthanasia solution such as pentobarbital, it will circulate throughout the body and cause changes, but one can avoid injecting near or into an organ of special interest. For example, if the cat is currently enrolled in a renal study, an intrarenal injection should not be performed. If a rabies test needs to be conducted, a physical method such as gunshot to the head should be avoided and so on. Laboratory researchers have a variety of euthanasia techniques that general practitioners do not use in private practice because of their need to preserve tissues. When possible, veterinarians can communicate with the place of study to determine which method of euthanasia is most appropriate.

## Inhalant methods

| Pros | Cons |
|------|------|
| • Cotton ball or gas machine | • Not ideal in the field |
| • Can induce death by itself | • Liquid form is corrosive |
| • No need for a needle injection | • Some gases are aversive |
| • Pre-euthanasia anesthesia too | • Risk of worker/onlooker inhalation |
| | • Poor uptake with respiratory disease |
| | • Some species are resistant |
| | • Gas cost and storage |
| | • Chambers create a physical barrier |

# Injectable methods

**Pros**
- Fast and effective
- Standard dosing
- +/− Sedation/anesthesia
- Minimal side effects

**Cons**
- Venous access typically necessary
- Blood pressure concerns
- Requires mild to advanced skill
- Most are controlled substances
- Unconsciousness required in some techniques
- Tissue residues

# Physical methods

**Pros**
- No tissue residue
- Fast and effective
- Relatively inexpensive to perform

**Cons**
- Requires specialized equipment
- Requires advanced training
- External bleeding is typical
- Secondary methods often needed
- Greater risk to personnel
- Increased risk of compassion fatigue

# Species-specific techniques

## Dogs and cats

The most common method of euthanasia in dogs and cats that are client owned, live within shelters, or in laboratories, is by injection of a barbiturate or barbiturate-combination solution. Typical inhalants are $CO_2$, CO, and anesthetics such as halothane and isoflurane. N and Ar are other inhalants that are used, but only in rare situations due to the availability of superior agents. In more extreme situations, other methods will be called upon that may be considered normal for other species. Examples of this include gunshot, injected anesthetics, or KCl injection.

### Inhalant agents

For client-owned dogs and cats, inhalant agents are rarely used to perform euthanasia. They are more commonly used in the shelter settings or for mass euthanasia. Whatever the situation, an ideal inhalant will be free of odor, nonirritating, and lead to rapid unconsciousness regardless of the size of the pet. The method in which it is delivered is also important. A device should be chosen with respect to the animal's comfort and familiarity whenever possible.

Any gas that is inhaled must reach a certain concentration in the alveoli before it can be effective (AVMA euthanasia guideline review 2011). Respiratory disease, anemia, and other diseases currently being experienced by the dog or cat may increase the time to unconsciousness and should be considered when choosing between an inhalant or injectable agent. Due to the superiority of other methods such as barbiturate injection, inhalant agents are generally reserved for puppies and kittens or in situations that require rapid, inexpensive depopulation such as in shelters.

If an inhalant agent must be used, the delivery method should be appropriate to the size and behavior of the animal. Dogs and cats less than 7 kg may be masked or placed in a chamber to receive the agent. Any dogs or cats larger than this would be unacceptable, according to the American Veterinary Medical Association (AVMA) unless a shelter situation negates it. If the animal is fractious, a chamber is preferred to avoid more handling than necessary. The chamber should meet the requirements listed in Chapter 2. Dogs and cats should be euthanized individually whenever possible, unless the veterinarian deems it appropriate to have two or more companions together for comfort. When unconsciousness is achieved, the gas may be used to complete death or another method may be performed.

## Noninhalant pharmaceutical agents
### Intravenous injection
In order to perform an IV euthanasia, the veterinarian or staff member will need to find a vein that can be injected with euthanasia solution. The accessory cephalic and cephalic veins in the front leg and the medial and lateral saphenous veins in the back leg are generally easy to see and feel. Each has its pros and cons. The administrator should pick the one that is most appropriate under the circumstances (see Table 5.1).

The veins themselves will be covered with the skin and usually lie on top of or in the grooves between neighboring muscles, tendons, and ligaments. Depending on the dog or cat, it may be necessary to first shave the intended area of injection. Shaving close to the skin provides a better view of the vein, thus minimizing multiple injection attempts (Rhoades 2002). If an awake pet does not like the sound of clippers, their use should be avoided or a pre-euthanasia sedative given to lessen distress.

The vein will need to be occluded by either a tourniquet or an assistant "holding off" the vein to build pressure distally. Occlusion of the vein should be done proximal to the injection site and with enough pressure that the vein can be easily seen and felt. In an awake animal, this should be done gently enough to avoid added stress. A socialized pet responds well to soft touches and supportive talking. If the vein cannot be easily seen or palpated, occlude again, gently squeezing the leg to increase venous blood return.

The lower on the limb the vein is, the more "roly-poly" it becomes. In general, the more proximal to the body, the more stable the vein becomes. This is due to the surrounding muscle bodies, fascia, etc. When choosing your injection site, consider skin diseases, masses, etc., that will make placement difficult.

When preparing to inject, either via direct venipuncture with a needle or with catheter use, hold the vein in place to minimize lateral movement. The

**Table 5.1** Common venous injection sites in dogs and cats.

**Lateral saphenous vein**
*Pros*
- Easy to locate
- Long length
- Away from the head where families like to gather
- Perfectly positioned when a pet is lying on its side

*Cons*
- Short legs make placement more difficult
- Poorer pressure due to distance from heart
- Loose skin, minimal fascia to hold the vein in place
- Vein can split into smaller veins

**Medial saphenous vein**
*Pros*
- Easy to locate
- Medium length
- Away from the head
- Body position builds blood volume in the vein

*Cons*
- Upper leg has to be moved out of the way
- Tourniquet placement more difficult
- Works better on cats than dogs

**Cephalic vein**
*Pros*
- Easy to locate
- Usually good diameter
- Long length
- Good pressures due to proximity to heart
- Consistent vein pattern

*Cons*
- Harder to place in lateral recumbency
- Near the head where families like to gather

cephalic vein can be supported on the side by the administrator's thumb. For the saphenous vein, which tends to be very movable, the administrator can secure the vein distal to the injection site using their thumb. Actually placing the thumb over the vein and applying a little tension distally will straighten out any kinks in the vein and tighten the skin. This essentially traps blood between the tourniquet and thumb, hopefully creating a nice target. Medial saphenous veins can be held in place by either technique. In general, keeping the skin tight over the injection site will also help anchor the vein and make injection easier. For direct venipuncture with euthanasia syringe and needle, the administrator should draw back and check for blood. To be safe, the administrator should do this at least once during venous administration to make sure that the needle is still placed correctly (see Figures 5.1-5.7).

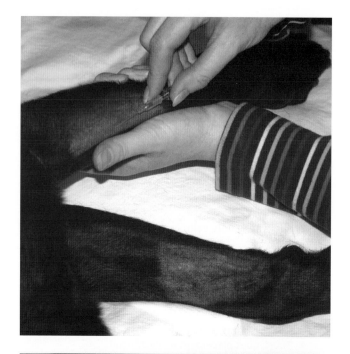

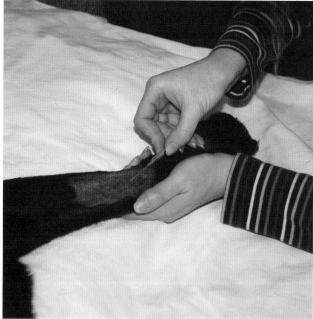

**Figure 5.1** Cephalic catheter placement in a dog.

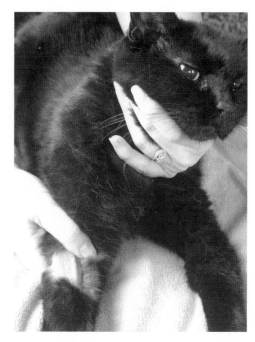

**Figure 5.2** Example of a highly visible cephalic vein in a cat after shaving.

More and more veterinary teaching institutions are recommending catheter placement for all IV euthanasia procedures. It is considered the gold standard for IV injections, even in sedated dogs and cats. Catheters help ensure that the euthanasia solution given will not accidentally be placed outside of the vein, as can happen with direct venipuncture. Direct venipuncture, either with

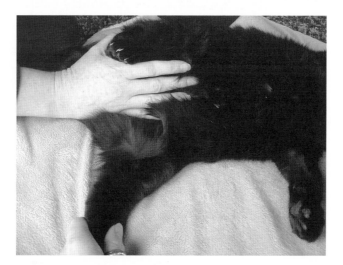

**Figure 5.3** Unshaved inner thigh hiding the medial saphenous vein in a cat. Note how hard it is to see the vein.

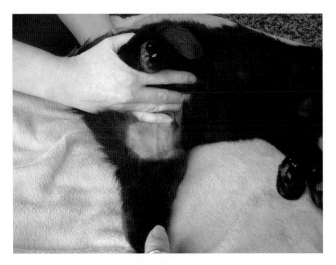

**Figure 5.4** Shaved inner thigh exposing medial saphenous vein in a cat.

a needle or butterfly catheter, creates a risk of the needle puncturing through the vein at any time. Catheter placement also opens up the option to offer the family some privacy before proceeding with the euthanasia (Cooney 2011). Catheters can be sealed with either a male adapter or extension set. An extension set is commonly used to allow the administrator to sit further back

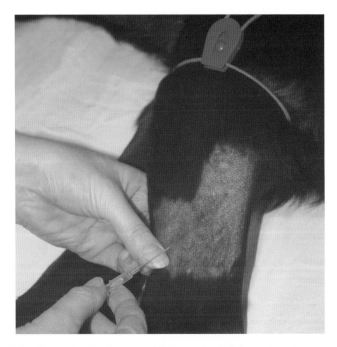

**Figure 5.5** Preparing to place a catheter in the left lateral saphenous vein in a dog.

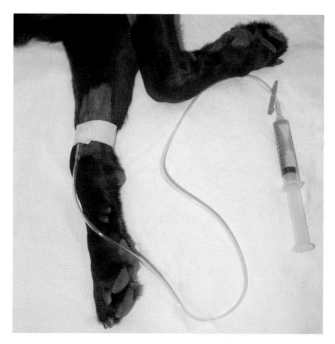

**Figure 5.6** Extension set with catheter in a dog.

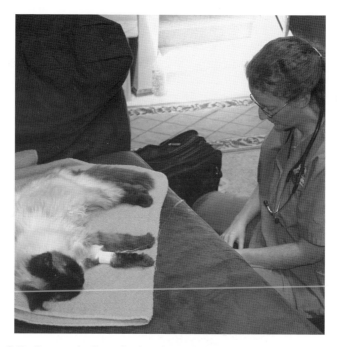

**Figure 5.7** Demonstration of extension set allowing the veterinarian to sit back and allow room for the client to gather close.

from the pet, giving more room for loved ones to gather close. Luer-locking mechanisms on either is recommended to help prevent leaking or dislodging of the syringe from the catheter hub. In the event of an emergency, a syringe with euthanasia solution may be directly connected to the catheter for more rapid administration.

If a good vein should "blow" at anytime during the initial catheter placement, injection, etc., it may still be possible to inject distally to the extravasation site, especially if the vein is highly visible there and moving to another leg will prove difficult. This location is not standard practice for a pet expected to survive, but when euthanasia is the objective, it is acceptable. Saline should be administered to check the new needle/catheter placement to see how much leakage there is at the original extravasation site. If there is little to none, which is usually the case, the euthanasia solution can be given while applying gentle pressure to the area. *Only attempt this if the pet is deeply sedated or completely anesthetized, due to the risk of pain from even slight euthanasia-solution extravasation.* Veterinarians should also inject more euthanasia solution than necessary due to this mild extravasation.

When families are present, the injection preparation can be a difficult time. They know that with every step completed, they are getting closer to the end. Offering reassuring words that things are proceeding as they should is helpful. If venous access is proving difficult, let those present know that everything is under control and their pet is doing fine. In this author's experience, families do not want to know technical details more than necessary. To avoid the technical portion, many clinics remove the pet back to the treatment area for catheter placement; however, this may disconnect the family and their pet at a very critical time. When possible, a technically skilled staff member or the veterinarian themselves should prepare the injection site in the room with family present. If they are interested in talking, ask them to tell a story about their pet. If they prefer quiet time for reflection, veterinarians and staff can continue in silence. In the case of a fractious pet that is reluctant to hold still for the injection, giving a pre-euthanasia sedative will make the process easier on everyone.

The standard barbiturate injection amount is 1 mL per 10 lb body weight for both dogs and cats. If the exact weight of the pet is unknown, make the best educated guess possible and give at least 2 mL more than the required amount (Cooney 2011). Giving more than recommended will hold true for any kind of euthanasia solution given. It also helps to have some extra euthanasia solution in the syringe in, case the drug leaks from a catheter set up, such as when a luer-lock is not securely fastened. If the euthanasia solution is extremely viscous, it can be diluted with saline to ease its movement through the needle and/or catheter.

Once the needle is inserted directly into the vein or a catheter is placed, inject slowly and steadily to avoid putting too much pressure on the area. When all of the solution has been properly injected, the needle or catheter may be removed. Apply pressure to the injection site to stop any bleeding. A catheter may be flushed with saline to clear any residual solution. The injection site should be checked to make sure there is no bleeding before allowing anyone to hold the body.

When performing an IV injection, death occurs very quickly. The onset of death with a barbiturate should be seen within 30 seconds or so (Fakkema 2008). KCl is also quick. As of 2011, overdoses of propofol or xylazine for euthanasia purposes have not been adequately studied and consistent time to death is unknown. Anyone present for the euthanasia should be told what to expect and how fast the death will occur. If the pet is sitting, it should be gently guided down toward the table or floor to avoid a rapid drop. In this author's experience, it is the sudden collapse that is most surprising to loved ones watching.

### Technical challenges

During the injection, there are a few scenarios that can occur leading to a less than perfect IV euthanasia. One such technically challenging scenario is the vein that cannot be found. Veins can be difficult to find for a variety of reasons: poor venous pressures, thickened or loose skin, improper tourniquet placement or handler's holding technique, poor lighting, etc. Those present to help with the euthanasia procedure should work together to prepare the site for injection. The administrator should be comfortable with the vein and only attempt injection when success is likely. If IV euthanasia of a dog or cat is being attempted by one person without assistance, pre-euthanasia sedation is strongly recommended, especially for fractious animals.

If a leg vein cannot be found, and IV euthanasia is the only acceptable method given the circumstances, a tongue vein or the jugular vein can be used. The tongue has multiple veins along the ventral surface, but one vein will likely be more prominent than the others. They can be occluded and stabilized similar to leg veins. Tongue veins should only be used in extreme situations, especially when family is present and given the personal nature of working in the pet's mouth. Because of the difficult location, all animals should be heavily sedated or anesthetized before attempting to inject a tongue vein. Jugular veins may also be used. Shaving the neck is encouraged to improve visibility. Depending on the dog or cat's neck structure, veins can be deep and difficult to palpate. Assistance is recommended when attempting to inject the jugular vein. A staff member or client can apply hand pressure near the thoracic inlet to improve vein size.

Another poor scenario is extravasation of the solution. If a bleb is seen forming in the surrounding tissue, the needle or catheter has slipped out of the vein. If the pet is fully sedated, there should not be any reaction. An awake animal will feel pain upon extravasation of the euthanasia solution. This is due to increased pressure within the subcutaneous (SQ) space and/or the chemical properties of the drug. The pet will likely vocalize or try to pull away from the injection site. A second injection attempt should be tried higher up the leg. What makes this scenario challenging is that the bleb makes placing a new injection proximally very difficult. The SQ bleb obscures the administrator's view of the original vein and may force the use of another one. Proceeding quickly helps keep the family comfortable and limits the time available for the misplaced injected solution to absorb and lower blood pressures. In the worst-case scenario of not being able to access a vein in another leg, the veterinarian will need to switch to another euthanasia method such as the IC or intra-abdominal injection.

Another difficult situation is when a catheter is placed within the vein, but the solution will not flow. Causes for this are a kinked catheter, a plug within the tip (either tissue or blood clot), or the tip pressed up against a venous valve or wall. When this happens, the catheter should be pulled out ever so slightly to see if flow resumes. If not, a new catheter will need to be placed proximally and the procedure started over.

If there is leakage around a properly placed catheter, the adaptor or extension has not been securely fastened together and solution is able to leak out. If this occurs, the setup should be examined and the problem corrected before proceeding. More solution may need to be drawn up if too much has leaked out and euthanasia cannot be achieved with the remaining amount.

Actively seizuring pets also pose a challenge. To place a catheter under these conditions, the administrator should use the leg that has the biggest vein or they feel most comfortable with. If someone is willing to help, they may steady the leg. With a back leg, they may push the stifle straight, and for the front leg, they can brace the elbow. Front legs tend to extend during seizures, which can be helpful when no one is available to assist. If the legs are paddling too much, the euthanasia injection may be administered into the heart or abdomen. IC injections are preferred because of their rapid action. Intra-abdominal absorption can take a long time and the pet will continue to seizure in the meantime.

Not having enough euthanasia solution may be the biggest technical challenge of all. This happens when the pet weighs more than anticipated, the pet is not passing normally and all remaining solution has been given, or inadequate volume of solution was available. Whatever the situation, it is important to find the next logical course of action to prevent suffering. If the inadequate amount is found before euthanasia is attempted, more solution should be acquired before proceeding. If the euthanasia procedure is in progress, an overdose of sedatives/anesthetics on hand, such as propofol, xylazine, or an inhalant gas such as isoflurane, can be administered. However, at this time, there are no scientific reports on the appropriate dosing of propofol, xylazine, or any other injectable anesthetic for euthanasia in dogs. One manufacturer of propofol gave an $LD_{50}$ of 30 mg/kg and suggested that 100 mg per 10 lb may be adequate for euthanasia. Something like this is only recommended in the direst of circumstances due to the availability of superior, more reliable, and inexpensive methods.

When no other drugs can be utilized, and euthanasia must be accomplished, a physical method will need to be attempted under anesthesia. If the euthanasia drug used was a barbiturate such as the common pentobarbital, a dose of

25-30 mg/kg IV may have already been given and is sufficient for anesthesia of dogs and cats (Plumb 2005). An example of this dose would be 1.5-2 mL of pentobarbital solution given IV to a 50-lb dog. Physical methods can then be attempted including gunshot, exsanguination, etc. Anyone present should be advised on the manner of death and reassured that their pet is free of pain and stressors.

### Intracardiac injection

Veterinary practitioners have performed IC injections for a very long time. Veterinarians choose cardiac sticks for a variety of reasons, most often when veins are not accessible or when an immediate death with little to no preparation is desirable, such as with a seizuring dog. However, no studies have ever been conducted comparing this method to other euthanasia techniques or to determine what depth of sedation is necessary for a dog or cat to be completely pain free. The challenge is to perform the procedure accurately, and when the family is present, perform it perfectly on the first attempt.

The simplest way to give an IC injection is to have the pet lying in lateral recumbency on either their right or left side. A pet lying on its right side is the standard position. The heart is easy to auscult from the left and the left ventricle is usually the easiest chamber to locate due to its size. The left side of the chest also has fewer lung lobes, but the right side does have the cardiac notch where no lung tissue resides. Heart and lung disease can complicate things; thickened myocardium, tumors, displacement, pulmonary edema/effusion, etc., even a large lipoma over the chest wall can make an IC injection difficult. In terms of death, there is little difference between using the right or left side of the heart. When injecting the right side, the right ventricular chamber is usually smaller than the left making injection more difficult. Once located however, time to cardiac arrest is essentially the same, even though solution from the right ventricle must pass through the lungs before making its way up to the brain.

A normal dog or cat will contain the following anatomical features that must be penetrated for a successful IC injection (from outside, moving in):

(1) Skin
(2) Body wall with costal musculature
(3) Costal pleura
(4) Pleural cavity
(5) Pericardial pleura–part of the mediastinal pleura
(6) Fibrous pericardium
(7) Serous pericardium
(8) Pericardial cavity
(9) Epicardium
(10) Myocardium
(11) Endocardium
(12) Ventricular chamber

If the lung is penetrated, the needle must pass through the pulmonary pleura and lung tissue itself.

The heart in most dogs and cats will reside from the 2nd or 3rd intercostal space (ICS) to the 5th or 6th ICS, and from the sternum to about two-thirds of the way up the thorax (Pasquini and Spurgeon 1992). In this author's experience, the heart is usually more cranial and ventral than one might think. When ausculting the heart, the administrator must pinpoint the PMI, or point of maximum intensity. On the left side of the chest, this will likely be the point of the aortic valve located in the 4th ICS at the level of the shoulder. On the right side, the right AV valve will generally be the loudest and is also in the 4th ICS at the level of the olecranon/elbow. The olecranon is located near the 5th ICS, so there will be little heart caudal to this point in a normal chest. A stethoscope or hand can be used to find the PMI on the chest wall. If necessary, the administrator can grasp the lower antebrachium and press the elbow up the chest wall to simulate where it would normally be if the dog or cat were standing. A good place to insert the needle is usually just a bit cranial to the point of the elbow. Combining the location of the PMI with this landmark should help locate the heart (Figures 5.8–5.10).

Before attempting an IC injection, all supplies should be ready to go before even locating the injection site. The animal must be completely unconscious and should not react in any way to the injection. When performing an IC injection in large dogs, a long needle will be required to reach the heart. Long needles, such as 1.5–2-in. needles can be used. Smaller dogs and cats will allow for shorter 1-in. needles. As the administrator prepares to enter the chest wall, the needle should be directed perpendicular to the body. Angling the needle will increase the distance needed to travel before locating the heart. If a rib is bumped during penetration of the chest wall, the administrator should either start over or gently walk the needle tip off the rib edge and keep going.

When the administrator believes the heart has been located, the syringe plunger can be withdrawn to check for blood. Proper placement leads to a rapid gush of blood. If only a small amount is found in the needle hub, the needle is within myocardium or small capillary. If negative pressure occurs within the syringe, the needle tip is within or against something solid (e.g., the myocardium, a tumor, a pleural lining, etc.). The needle should be advanced further and aspiration attempted again. If blood is still not found, the administrator can gently redirect without removing the needle completely from the chest.

A large syringe, with extra room for aspiration, should be used to hold the solution. When injecting into the heart, the administrator will draw back blood to make sure they are within a chamber, and therefore, a little extra room in the syringe is necessary. If giving 6 mL of solution, this author recommends using a 12-ml syringe rather than a 6-ml syringe. Blood, pulmonary fluid, and air can be aspirated into the syringe. Once obvious blood is in the syringe, the administrator is free to inject the euthanasia solution. It is always good practice to draw back again halfway through the injection to check for proper

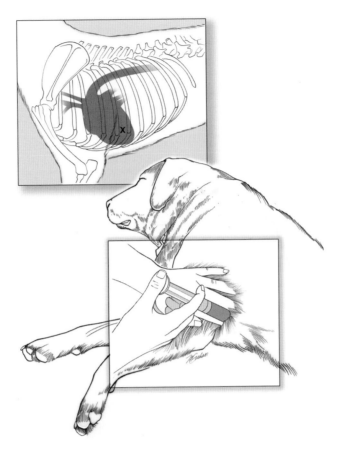

**Figure 5.8** Proper placement of intracardiac injection in the left side of a dog.

placement. When all of the solution has entered the heart, death should occur quickly.

Administering more solution than required is good practice with IC injections (Cooney 2011). If the pet weighs 40 lb, and the solution dose is 1 mL per 10 lb, administering at least 6 mL will help ensure that death takes place. There is no limit to how much solution can be given with any technique. A higher volume allows for minor accidental injection outside of the heart, which is never ideal, but does commonly occur.

When the administrator is holding the syringe in the heart, it may move along with the contractions. This is disturbing for any loved ones present to see, so the syringe should never be let go. A free hand can be used to shield the syringe from view if necessary. When properly performed, the IC injection is no more invasive than any other technique; however, those present should be prepared for what they will witness. If anyone expresses concern, the veterinarian's hand or a drape of some sort can be placed to limit visibility (Figure 5.11).

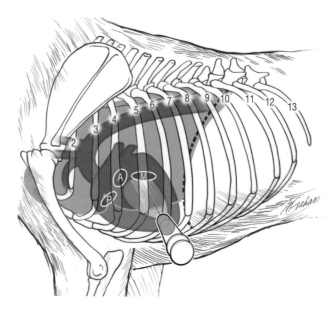

**Figure 5.9** Anatomical landmarks for left-sided cardiac injection in dogs.

Before performing an IC injection, the administrator may need to share with the family why this method is best for their pet. In this author's experience, some families have found it difficult to watch and accept, especially when proven to be technically challenging. When the pet is unconscious, this technique remains one of the most efficient methods used today.

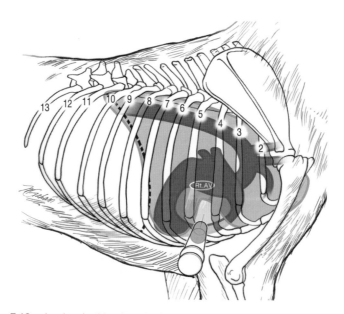

**Figure 5.10** Anatomical landmarks for right-sided cardiac injection in dogs.

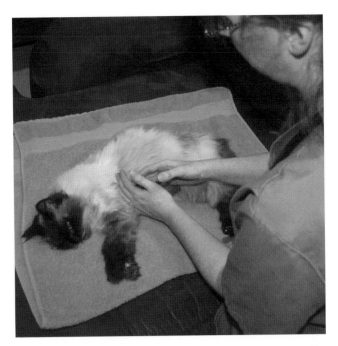

**Figure 5.11** Veterinarian's hand shielding visibility of the intracardiac injection.

### Technical challenges

Due to the higher level of skill required to perform IC injections, more technical challenges present. The administrator cannot see the heart itself, so the injection site is based solely on anatomical landmarks and auscultation. What exactly lies beneath the chest wall can only be learned once the technique is started. Ultrasound or radiography might be used to increase visibility.

If pulmonary effusion/edema is present, pulmonary fluid may be aspirated before blood. Having extra room in the syringe will allow the administrator to redirect and try again without having to draw up a new syringe full of euthanasia solution. The same holds true for air aspirated from lung tissue, airways, etc.

When the heart is difficult to locate, and the syringe is full of fluid (both solution and pulmonary fluid) or air, the syringe can be gently expressed in the chest. If this does not seem like a viable option, the administrator can express the contaminated syringe contents into a towel or trash container and redraw fresh solution to start again. Injecting a small to moderate amount of euthanasia solution into the chest of an unconscious animal should not have any adverse effects, especially when euthanasia can still be quickly carried out (Cooney 2011). All wasted drug will need to be recorded.

There will be times when the heart is impossible to find; the chest is too deep, the needle length is inadequate, the heart is not in the standard position due to disease, etc. When the heart cannot be located, it will become necessary to attempt another technique altogether. When loved ones are present, multiple

IC needle insertions are not advised. Another technique should be attempted as soon as it becomes evident that the heart cannot be found.

In the rare instance when ample blood is in the syringe and the solution is injected successfully, but the pet is not passing, the solution has been third-spaced somewhere. The solution is possibly trapped in the pericardial cavity or some other blood-filled space and cannot make its way to the brainstem. At this point, the administrator should attempt another cardiac injection or move to another location such as the liver.

Sometimes, pushing down on the needle during injection will move it out of the ventricular chamber. A steady hand is needed throughout the injection. If the needle moves out of the chamber during injection, the needle should first be redirected to locate it again. If blood cannot be found, the contents of the syringe can be expressed within the chest and the procedure immediately started again.

### Intraperitoneal injection

An IP injection is generally considered easier to perform than most other methods. It is a nice alternative to IV injections when poor venous pressures are observed. The euthanasia solution is given into the peritoneal space, that is, the abdomen. Therefore, the solution must miss neighboring organs or the administration would be considered intraorgan, which without anesthesia is considered painful. IP injections are very common and work on all domesticated cats and dogs, including young kittens and puppies. Fetal euthanasia is also commonly achieved via this method following the removal of the uterus from the bitch or queen.

Shelters in particular use this technique on a daily basis due to the low level of skill required to perform them and that no sedation is required for pure sodium pentobarbital administration. According to the 2012 AMVA euthanasia guidelines, only pure barbiturates are approved for IP injection in awake animals. Barbiturate-combination drugs, such as Beuthanasia-D® from Schering-Plough, are only approved through IV or IC injection because of the added component phenytoin sodium. Should phenytoin sodium be absorbed first, leading to premature cardiac arrest before pentobarbital-induced unconsciousness, the animal may experience distress. Please refer to the drug reference sheet for all approved solution administration sites.

There are two approved sites of IP injection: (1) ventral midline caudal to the umbilicus and (2) low on the right lateral abdomen (Rhoades 2002). These locations prove most reliable for avoiding abdominal organs. Smaller needle length such as 0.75–1 in. is recommended to avoid deeper organs. If the body wall is abnormally thickened, a longer needle should be used. To minimize pain, the needle bore size should be appropriate to the size of the animal and the solution given at a rate of 1 mL/s. Newborns handle 25-gauge, 5/8-in. needles well, and obese cats up to 20-gauge, 1-in. needles (see Figure 5.12; Fakkema 2008).

The needle should be inserted at an angle slightly toward the head and the syringe plunger pulled to check for fluid. If no blood or fluid is seen in the syringe, the administrator may inject the solution. Because the euthanasia

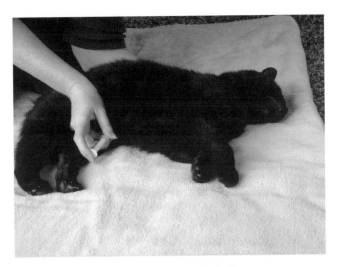

**Figure 5.12** Cat receiving an intraperitoneal injection.

solution is moving into the blood stream through absorption across abdominal organ membranes and serosal linings, it may take longer to achieve cardiac death. An awake pet may take up to 10-15 minutes to reach unconsciousness with another 5-10 minutes before cardiac arrest (Rhoades 2002). It may take this long or longer for a sedated pet to die due to lowered blood pressures. When necessary, the abdomen can be gently massaged to help the solution absorb.

Dogs and cats that are not pre-sedated should be placed in quiet rooms, cages, etc., free of distraction. This will allow a smoother transition into unconsciousness. The animal may paddle, appear disoriented, lick their lips, and vocalize a bit as the drug starts to take effect. These movements correlate to Stages 1 and 2 of anesthesia (Fakkema 2008). If the owner is present, they can hold the pet offering comfort, but due to the unpredictable nature of Stage 1 and 2 anesthesia, risk of personal injury should be considered. Pre-euthanasia sedation/anesthesia might be warranted when owners are present. In this author's experience, sedation does not appear to greatly increase time to cardiac arrest.

IP injections require the administration of more barbiturate solution than the standard 1 mL per 10 lb. The recommended dose is 3 mL per 10 lb. If more than one injection is needed when family is present, the family can be updated on why more is being given. Because waiting for a pet to die can be difficult for some, injecting an area of high perfusion such as the liver or kidney under anesthesia is recommended over the standard IP injection. Death must be verified closely to make sure deep unconsciousness is not confused with death and the pet subsequently recovers.

### Technical challenges

There has been discussion on the validity of this technique without pre-euthanasia sedation/anesthesia due to the possibility of abdominal irritation from barbiturate injection. Specifically, a study looking at abdominal irritation in rats following barbiturate injection demonstrated tissue irritation (Wadham 1997). If subsequent studies demonstrate consistent findings, pre-euthanasia sedation/anesthesia may be required for all IP injections using pure barbiturates. As of 2011, Vortech Pharmaceuticals is working on FDA approval of a new barbiturate-combination drug (FP-3®) containing lidocaine. This solution works by eliminating pain at the injection and absorption site. If effective, FP-3 may be an ideal IP injection solution for awake or sedated pets. Until a combination product like this is marketed, local anesthetics may also be given to lessen pain at the injection site.

Based on the speed of abdominal absorption, it is possible for this technique to take up to an hour or more before death is achieved. Abdominal fluid, weak blood pressures, and simply third spacing can all contribute to the rate of absorption. When these factors are taken into consideration, IP injections may not be the best technique to use.

This technique requires specific solution to be given in an awake animal. Pre-euthanasia anesthesia must be given when administering a barbiturate-combination drug. Anesthetic overdoses with propofol, xylazine, etc., are not appropriate for IP injections. Pure barbiturates are the only drug allowed for this technique. More solution must be administered to avoid deep unconsciousness without cardiac arrest.

If an organ is injected in an awake pet, the pet will likely squirm and try to move away from the handler. The injection should be stopped and redirected. If all the available solution has been given, and the pet has not died within a reasonable amount of time, more solution should be quickly acquired before the pet regains consciousness or a physical method of euthanasia should be performed.

### Intrahepatic injection

The liver is large, highly vascular, and is usually easy to palpate. Veterinarians choose intrahepatic injections over intra-abdominal injections because of the improved uptake of the euthanasia solution, especially when clients are present. This organ resides right up against the diaphragm and for the most part, takes up to half of the caudal rib cage space. Seated within its curvature will be the stomach, gall bladder, and proximal small intestine. When an IV injection is not viable, an intrahepatic injection can be a great alternative (Cooney 2011).

Like IC injections, intrahepatic injections need to be done in unconscious pets. They may cause pain in an awake pet due to parenchymal swelling and possible irritation from the euthanasia solution. Before injecting the liver, absence of deep pain and reflexes should be checked; pinch the toes, touch around the eye, etc. When no response is seen, the administrator is safe to inject. Because the pet is unconscious, it will likely be laterally recumbent making hepatic injection easier.

A needle long enough to reach the liver should be used. With small pets, a 1-in. needle should be adequate, but in larger pets, a 1.5- or 2-in. needle may

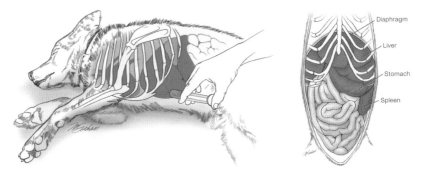

**Figure 5.13** Anatomical landmarks for intrahepatic injections in dogs and cats.

be necessary. To inject the liver, the needle will have to be placed in the notch on either side of the xyphoid process or wherever a liver lobe can be easily palpated (Figure 5.13). The liver is best reached by aiming cranially, up under the last rib of the laterally recumbent pet. Inward pressure with the syringe or with the administrator's free hand will allow the needle to move deeper. Aspirating and detecting blood usually indicates the needle is correctly placed; however, absence of blood does not mean the placement is wrong. Intrahepatic injections are effective from either the left or right side of the body (Figure 5.14).

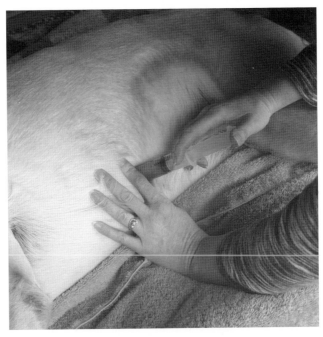

**Figure 5.14** Injection in the left side of the liver in a dog. Note this dog's liver could be palpated easily in this region.

Intrahepatic injections require the administration of more barbiturate solution than the standard 1 mL per 10 lb. The recommended dose is 2 mL per 10 lb (Cooney 2011). If more than one injection is needed when family is present, the they can be updated on why more is being given. Death should occur within about 2 minutes or so with a well-performed intrahepatic injection (Grier and Schaffer 1990; Cooney 2011). Cessation of breathing should be almost immediate. In case the injection does not entirely penetrate the liver, anyone present should be prepared that death may take up to 10 minutes or more.

### Technical challenges

If the administrator feels the liver was not injected properly, death may not occur in a reasonable amount of time and more solution should be given, especially when loved ones are present. A second full dose of solution may be injected toward the liver again or placed in another area of high perfusion such as a kidney. If the second injection is given and the pet continues to breathe, the administrator may gently massage the region to increase blood flow and absorption time. When cardiac death takes longer than 10 minutes, either an IP injection was performed or the area of liver injected was not well perfused. If all the available solution has been given, and the pet has not died within a reasonable amount of time, more solution should be quickly acquired before the pet regains consciousness or a physical method of euthanasia performed. Good planning will help to prevent this.

### Intrarenal injections

Intrarenal injections are a viable option for cats and small mammals. This method is a great choice if venous access is difficult or when preparing a catheter site is too obtrusive. This technique is noninvasive and works well when loved ones are present. They can easily hold the pet on their lap keeping the human–animal bond strong. As with intrahepatic injections, renal tissue will improve the rate of absorption over standard IP injections. Complete unconsciousness is required to attempt this technique. For instructional purposes here, this technique will be demonstrated in cats.

Feline kidneys and kidneys of small mammals are usually easy to palpate, especially if the animal has a normal to poor body condition score. The kidneys are a paired structure lying adjacent to the sublumbar muscles alongside the vertebral column. Increased abdominal fat decreases the administrator's ability to isolate either kidney. Assuming both kidneys are present, the administrator will be able to choose the most appropriate one to inject.

In general, the right kidney will reside more cranially than the left. It is usually located just under the last two ribs along the dorsum. The left kidney in contrast is more caudal and free of the overlying ribs. In cats, the left kidney rests outside the retroperitoneal space making it easier to isolate than the right.

When choosing which kidney to inject, the administrator can use the one they feel and isolate the best. This author, being right-handed, prefers to use the left kidney. If a cat is in renal failure, the kidneys may be smaller, have a nodular feeling, or even be impossible to locate. Abdominal masses or fecal

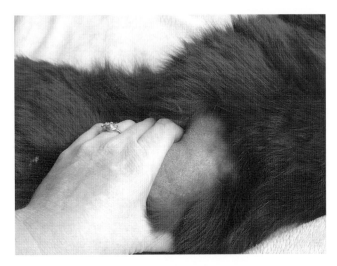

**Figure 5.15** Cupping the kidney in a cat (shaved for added visualization only).

balls in the colon are sometimes confused with kidneys. Should one kidney be assessed as unusable, the other may be tried.

Once the feline patient is completely anesthetized, it should be laid in a lateral recumbent position either on a table, owner's lap, etc. The administrator will move their hands along the abdomen to find the kidney and feel for any abdominal muscle tensing. If the cat tenses, it is not yet in a surgical plane of anesthesia and ready for injection. If necessary, more pre-euthanasia anesthesia will need to be given until no response. For left kidney injections, the cat should be positioned on its right side with legs facing away from the administrator. For right kidney injections, the cat should be down on the left side and a finger used to draw the kidney caudally from under the ribs. The right kidney will shift by only a centimeter or two.

When ready for euthanasia, the administrator may likely need to use both hands to gently isolate the kidney before switching to one hand to hold it in place. From the cat's downside, a hand can help to push the kidney upward for easier grasping. Once within reach, the administrator's less dominant hand can cup the kidney within their fingertips raising it up as far dorsal as possible (Figure 5.15).

If this cupping motion proves too challenging due to abdominal fat, scar tissue, etc., the kidney can be trapped firmly in a position by pressing the index finger and middle finger at each renal pole. The kidney will need to be held in place throughout the entire injection. When loved ones are present, any manipulation of the abdomen should be subtle.

To inject, the administrator will hold the syringe alongside the body directed toward the dorsum (see Figure 5.16). A 1-in. needle length of 18-22 gauge should be sufficient to easily penetrate the kidney. Diseased kidneys can feel granular, cystic, etc., making needle insertion more difficult. The syringe can be shielded from view by tucking it below the hand holding the kidney. This is a very effective way to hide the injection from onlookers. If the kidney is located

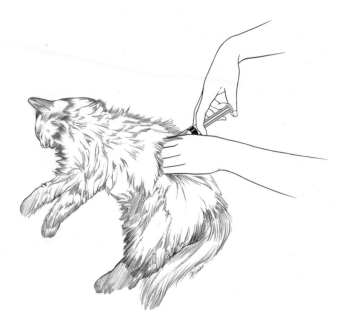

**Figure 5.16** Demonstration of intrarenal injection in a cat.

deep in the abdomen, the syringe will have to be held more perpendicular to the body.

The needle should be inserted deep within the renal parenchyma, avoiding the renal pelvis (Figure 5.17). Injecting the pelvis may move the euthanasia solution into the ureter, limiting absorption. The kidney is a highly perfused organ, as one might expect based on its function, making it an ideal organ for rapid uptake of solution.

As this technique is considered relatively new, there remains no standardization of euthanasia solution dosing; however, barbiturates are the only type of drug used. Private practitioner reports indicate that anywhere from 2 mL per 10 lb up to 6 mL total per cat is effective with a properly executed injection. This author administers 6 mL per cat with excellent results. Whatever the volume, the kidney may swell due to increased pressure within the renal capsule. This is a good indication that the needle is positioned properly within the renal cortex. Kidney swelling does not guarantee immediate death, but it does increase the odds that death will occur faster (Cooney 2011). A proper injection within a viable kidney should produce respiratory and cardiac arrest within 30 seconds or so. Depending on the volume of solution given, the cat may pass before completing the injection. As with intrahepatic injections, loved ones present should be informed their pet may pass immediately or within just a few minutes.

### Technical challenges
A common technical challenge with intrarenal injections is losing hold of the kidney. If the administrator inadvertently lets go of the kidney mid-injection,

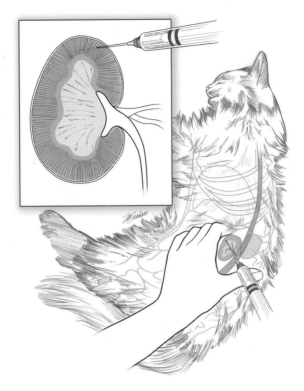

**Figure 5.17** Anatomical landmarks for intrarenal injections in cats.

and it cannot be quickly isolated again, the needle can be gently advanced toward the liver and the injection finished. This may not be necessary if the majority of the solution was administered before the kidney was lost. However, giving the remaining solution into an area of high perfusion helps to guarantee a more rapid death.

Another challenge is the absence of the administrator's preferred kidney. Many older pets, cats in particular, have small to nonexistent kidneys on one side making injection more difficult, especially when moving the pet is not an option with loved ones present. It can be awkward to roll a pet over onto its other side when an owner is holding it close. An example of this is the left kidney missing from a cat lying on its right side. The right kidney must now be used. If the right kidney cannot be fully grasped while the cat is lying on its right side, it can be isolated using the index and middle finger from the administrator's nondominant hand. These two fingers will essentially "trap" the kidney in place for injection.

Some well-placed intrarenal injections will result in prolonged time to cardiac death. Reasons for this prolonged time may include poor venous pressures, injection of a diseased kidney, or injection into an area of minimal vasculature such as the renal pelvis. These reasons are pure speculations as no scientific studies have been conducted to date. Whatever the reason behind the prolonged time, there are ways to compensate. If the administrator has injected the full dose, and the pet is still breathing, a repeat injection may be given immediately following. When the family is present, the second injection can be explained as "giving the rest." In general, when administering any type of euthanasia solution with any method other than IV injection, loved ones present can be prepared for up to two injections. When one injection is not achieving death in a timely manner, a second can always be given. In the case of intrarenal injections, this author immediately administers a second full dose whenever breathing continues following the first injection. The second injection may be directed toward the same kidney, assuming it is viable, or injected deeper internally. However, the spleen may be best to avoid since splenic injection may lead to slower uptake (Grier and Schaffer 1990). Based on preliminary findings from a retrospective study in 2012 on intrarenal injections in cats, a second injection within an area of high perfusion should lead to cardiac death within 2 minutes.

### Oral administration

Euthanasia through oral barbiturate administration is not common practice in the United States. When necessary, as in the case of feral or aggressive dogs or cats that pose risk to human safety, barbiturates can be given in powder form within food or liquid squirted into the mouth. The purpose of this method is to distance the animal from human contact as much as possible to limit injury. Oral administration may be used if needles or pre-euthanasia sedatives/anesthetics are unavailable. If unconsciousness can be achieved through oral dosing, a secondary method of euthanasia may be employed that is more reliable.

If liquid solution is given orally, three times the normal IV dose must be ingested for death to be achieved. This means a 50-lb dog needs 15 mL for death. A 10-lb cat will need 3 mL for death. Based on the dosage of 25–30 mg/kg for barbiturate-induced anesthesia, a 50-lb dog will need to receive 1.5-2 mL orally just to lose consciousness. Since barbiturates are poor tasting, proper administration of them in a liquid form is difficult and true ingestion becomes hard to determine. If liquid is to be given orally, the pet may need to have its mouth pried open, which can cause stress. In the case of extremely aggressive animals, it can be squirted through cage walls into the mouth of a barking dog, a hissing cat, etc.

Powdered forms of barbiturates are also available in the market and appear to be more reliable for effective dosing (Fakkema 2008). Fatal Plus® powder from Vortech is the only barbiturate powder approved for oral administration. The powder must be placed within food or within gelatin capsules for consumption. The correct dosing can be found in Table 5.2.

According to the American Humane Association's Euthanasia Training Guide, an animal receiving adequate oral dosing of a barbiturate should be in Stage 3 of anesthesia within 40 minutes of ingestion and dead within 2 hours. Times will vary depending on overall health of the animal, the rate of absorption, environmental stimulation, and so on. Whenever possible, the animal should be kept in a quiet, dark space to encourage relaxation and limit

Table 5.2  Oral dosage chart.

| Weight | | Species | Liquid | Amount of powder | | | 5 grain/capsule | Presentation | |
|---|---|---|---|---|---|---|---|---|---|
| lb | kg | Example | ml | Grains | mg | g | | Teaspoon | Tablespoon |
| 1.5 | 0.68 | Kitten (6 week) | 1.0 | 6 | 390 | 0.39 | 1 | 1/10 | |
| 2 | 0.9 | Kitten (8 week) | 1.0 | 6 | 390 | 0.39 | 1 | 1/10 | |
| 3 | 1.4 | Kitten (12 week) | 1.0 | 6 | 390 | 0.39 | 1 | 1/10 | |
| 8 | 3.6 | Cat | 3.0 | 18 | 1,170 | 1.17 | 4 | 1/4 | |
| 10 | 4.5 | Puppy (8 week) | 3.0 | 18 | 1,170 | 1.17 | 4 | 1/4 | |
| 15 | 6.8 | Cairn Terrier | 4.5 | 27 | 1,755 | 1.76 | 5 | 1/2 | |
| 20 | 9.1 | Fox Terrier | 6.0 | 36 | 2,340 | 2.34 | 7 | 1/2 | |
| 25 | 11.4 | Beagle | 7.5 | 45 | 2,925 | 2.93 | 9 | 3/4 | 1/4 |
| 30 | 13.6 | Cocker Spaniel | 9.0 | 54 | 3,510 | 3.51 | 11 | 3/4 | 1/4 |
| 40 | 18.2 | Springer Spaniel | 12.0 | 72 | 4,680 | 4.68 | 14 | 1 | 1/3 |
| 50 | 22.7 | Irish Setter | 15.0 | 90 | 5,850 | 5.85 | 18 | 1 1/2 | 1/2 |
| 60 | 27.3 | Labrador | 18.0 | 108 | 7,020 | 7.02 | 22 | 1 1/2 | 1/2 |
| 70 | 31.8 | Airedale | 21.0 | 126 | 8,190 | 8.19 | 25 | 2 | 3/4 |
| 80 | 36.4 | German Shepherd | 24.0 | 144 | 9,360 | 9.36 | 29 | 2 | 3/4 |
| 90 | 40.9 | Rottweiler | 27.0 | 162 | 10,530 | 10.53 | 32 | 2 1/2 | 3/4 |
| 100 | 45.4 | Great Dane | 30.0 | 180 | 11,700 | 11.70 | 36 | 2 3/4 | 1 |
| 150 | 68.2 | Mastiff | 45.0 | 270 | 17,550 | 17.55 | 54 | 3 1/2 | 1 1/2 |
| 200 | 90.9 | St. Bernard | 60.0 | 360 | 23,400 | 23.40 | 72 | 5 | 2 |

*Source:* Vortech® Pharmaceuticals, Ltd. 7/95
*Weight:* 1 kg equals 2.2 lb.
*Solution:* liquid dosage is calculated on 390 mg/ml or 6 grains/ml.
*Record keeping:* subtract the amount of powder removed in grams.
*Presentation:* number of capsules, based on 5 grains per capsule.
Amount per teaspoon is based on approximately 4.5 g per teaspoon. Amount per tablespoon is based on approximately 13 g per tablespoon.

stimulation. The animal will move slowly through Stages 1 and 2 of anesthesia and exhibit unpredictable behaviors. Animals should remain undisturbed during this time until full unconsciousness is observed, that is, no response to sound, gentle touches, lack of reflexes, etc. Euthanasia by oral administration of a barbiturate is very unreliable and the administrator should never assume that death has occurred, even if all of the drug was properly consumed. Verification of death must be done before disposing of the body.

### Technical challenges

The most obvious technical challenge is the inability to have the pet ingest the drug when placed in food. If the pet is friendly and responsive to people, soft soothing talk may help facilitate ingestion. For those more averse to human contact, stepping away from the area may make the pet feel safer and facilitate ingestion. Lightly heating the food may increase the release of aromas and stimulate appetite.

When the plan is to squirt it into the pet's mouth, timing will be very important. If the solution misses the mouth and is wasted, another attempt can be tried or a different method may need to be done. Barbiturates such as pentobarbital are very alkalinic and foul tasting, which even the gentlest of pets will dislike. Unfortunately, the easiest way to squirt drug into a fractious pet's mouth is when it is hissing or barking at the administrator. This indicates that the pet is angry or in distress, which is not an ideal euthanasia situation, but may be necessary for death to be achieved.

### Physical methods

There are only a few acceptable and conditionally acceptable physical methods of euthanasia available for dogs and cats. These methods, considered unpleasant to watch and perform, should only be used when injectable agents cannot be used for whatever reason. They will only be briefly addressed due to the infrequency of their use in private practice. Due to obvious reasons, these are not acceptable methods of euthanasia in dogs and cats when owners are present unless pronounced suffering necessitates their use.

### Gunshot

Euthanasia by gunshot is considered conditionally acceptable in dogs and cats in the 2012 AVMA guidelines. There are other, more reliable methods of euthanasia and these should always be considered first before resorting to gunshot use. If attempted, the pet should be quieted as much as possible. Due to the requirement for preciseness of the shot, fractious pets should be completely restrained using muzzles, cat bags, large blankets, etc., to render them immobilized. This will not only keep the handler safe, but help guarantee the gunshot is properly performed. Whenever possible, pets should be sedated or anesthetized to calm them and minimize movements, especially for cats and their smaller forehead size (Longair et al. 1991). If the pet is out of reach, and cannot be sedated using oral sedatives in food, highly skilled personnel will be required to perform the shot at a distance.

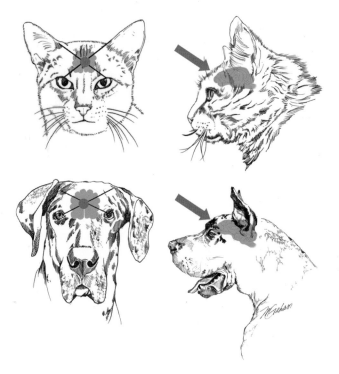

**Figure 5.18** Anatomical landmarks for gunshot or captive bolt use in dogs and cats.

Euthanasia by gunshot can be accomplished with a variety of firearms. If the approach is made within 3 ft of the pet, handguns or small caliber rifles are preferred. Close-range shooting is commonly performed with .22-caliber rifle or handgun or .410-gauge shotgun with slugs or pellets within 1-2 in. of the skull (Longair et al. 1991). Longer range attempts up to 2 m or so can be accomplished with a .308 rifle or larger gauge shotgun. The farther the distance from the dog or cat, the greater the risk of improper placement. This will endanger not only the pet, but also those gathered nearby.

Whether the pet is standing or lying down, the gun will be aimed directly toward the rostral forehead, as seen in Figure 5.18. The bullet should travel directly through the forehead into the brain with continuation down into the neck whenever possible. This prevents the bullet from leaving the body, putting others in harm's way, and directs it through the region of the brainstem causing instant unconsciousness and death. This method is standard for all domestic animals, except those with horns.

In dogs, the firearm is aimed at the point midway between the level of the eyes and ears. Some literature suggests aiming slightly off to one side to miss the thick midline bony ridge. With respect to the ears, the lines should be drawn to the dorsal medial edge closest to the medial plane. Because dogs have many different ear types, the shooter will have to use their best judgment. Imaginary crossing lines can be visualized from the ear to the medial canthus of the opposite eye. Again, the angle should be such that the bullet passes through the brain into the neck. To help position the dog perfectly and keep it relatively still, food may be placed in front on something elevated. This elevation will keep the neck parallel to the ground. In lying dogs, the gun should be aimed the same.

For cats, the gunshot technique should only be used in the most extreme of circumstances. Pre-euthanasia sedation is highly recommended to limit free movement of the head. Fractious cats can also be offered food to help them hold still, but they may need to be restrained. Restricting movement for any animal being euthanized is not ideal as this will cause stress and anxiety, but it may need to be done when aiming at a small target such as a cat's forehead. The firearm should be aimed at the center of the cat's head slightly below a line drawn connecting the base of the ears.

Instant unconsciousness and death is the goal with this physical method. Even with properly executed shots, the pet's body may spasm for a short while and bleeding will occur (Longair et al. 1991). Any one watching should be prepared for these physical signs and reassured that they are purely involuntary and that death was accomplished.

### Technical challenges

The reason this method is deemed conditionally acceptable and only to be used in the most specific of circumstances owes to the technical challenges it presents. The pet must be perfectly positioned or the bullet will miss the brainstem and put the pet at risk for pain and distress. Bullets can do remarkable damage to the head of a small animal and onlookers will likely find the technique disturbing to watch. If the bullet misses the brainstem, the administrator will need to fire another better placed shot. If only one bullet was available, and the pet is now suffering, blunt force trauma or some other physical method to the head may be necessary to speed death. Again, this is assuming that an acceptable method of euthanasia was never an option. Gunfire is also very loud and may cause stress to other animals gathered around.

### Penetrating captive bolt

The frequency of the usage of this technique is not known and it is only approved for use in dogs, not cats. When inhalant or injectable agents cannot be used, and other physical methods do not meet the requirements for death, such as in tissue sampling for laboratory medicine, this technique may be applied. The penetrating captive bolt technique may be used by itself to accomplish death. No other technique will need to be used secondarily unless signs of death are uncertain and the attending veterinary feels another method needs to be used.

Captive bolt guns can be used on dogs in any position, keeping in mind that the body will drop rapidly to the ground. Dogs euthanized in lateral recumbency eliminate this falling motion. The dog should be calmed naturally with soothing talk, offered food, or pre-sedated to minimize movement of the head. The bolt gun is placed centered in the forehead exactly like the gunshot location. Typical bolt guns fire a .22 caliber blank to mobilize the rod out of the barrel to penetrate the forehead. For best penetration, the end of the barrel should rest against the skin, be aimed toward the medulla oblongata, and trigger pulled for rod penetration into the skull (Dennis and Dong 1988). Brain disruption, including the medulla oblongata, is needed to achieve immediate unconsciousness and death.

Upon successful captive bolt usage, the dog will have immediate cerebral death and respiratory arrest, and cardiac arrest due to anoxia within 5 minutes (Dennis and Dong 1988). Some objectionable side effects such as extensor rigidity, reflexive movements, and urination/defecation may make the technique difficult to watch, but based on study results, all movements appear to be involuntary. The bolt will carry skin, debris, and bone into the head, so brain tissue sampling is not recommended with this method. The procedure is safer than the gunshot technique when observers are present. There is no bullet that could ricochet and cause injury.

### Technical challenges

Captive bolt guns have a tendency to fail when not properly maintained (Grandin 1998). The bolt will become covered in blood and tissue following use, and therefore, must be thoroughly cleaned after each euthanasia. Captive bolt guns are also loud and may cause distress to other animals in the area.

Should the placement of the gun be incorrect, the bolt will not penetrate the brainstem. This may lead to pain and distress if unconsciousness has not been achieved. Another firing will have to be done. If the bolt is not long enough to penetrate the brainstem, a pithing rod will be needed to disrupt the tissue. This is considered extremely unpleasant to do and should be avoided if at all possible by having a bolt long enough to complete death.

### Exsanguination

The goal of exsanguination is to rapidly deplete the brain and heart of oxygen causing rapid death. Exsanguination is considered an adjunctive method of euthanasia in unconscious dogs and cats, but is rarely ever done due to the availability of more acceptable methods. It is considered unacceptable when owners are present unless severe suffering warrants it and they agree to its use.

Exsanguination should be done using a very sharp knife, with at least a 6-in. rigid blade. These specifications come from what this author knows of goat exsanguination protocols for military personnel survival training. The knife is thrust into the neck just below the head, ventral to the vertebrae and drawn downward to sever the jugular veins, carotid arteries, and trachea. Blood should be directed toward a drain or depression in the ground. For sanitary reasons, it should be completely cleaned up before other animals are allowed in the area. When a client must be present, it may be advisable to attempt an internal cut of the myocardium to allow blood to flow into the chest cavity rather than out on the ground. To date, there is no scientific data to demonstrate this technique or support its reliability.

Exsanguination is rarely considered in dogs and cats due to the availability of superior methods and is only mentioned here to offer yet another possibility for use in dire situations. It is technically challenging in and of itself to safely penetrate the neck with a knife and sever it across laterally. Muscle, ligaments, nerves, and the trachea make a smooth sweeping motion almost impossible. More often than not, as demonstrated with goat slaughter training videos, there must be a sawing-like motion to perform adequate exsanguination.

The amount of blood released also poses a technical challenge. Visibility while cutting is reduced and it will contaminate everything around the body. There must be a cleanup plan to remove all blood.

### Blunt force trauma

This physical action is rarely effective in causing death by itself and is considered a conditionally acceptable method in neonates. It more commonly causes stunning and unconsciousness and is then followed by a secondary method of euthanasia. Mature craniums are designed to withstand head injuries, and therefore, very strong force is needed to disrupt the central nervous system (AVMA euthanasia guideline review 2011). It is most appropriate for neonatal animals with thin skull bones. This method can produce acceptable euthanasia when the blow provides sufficient force to cause a depressed fracture of the skull and physical damage to the brain. Any instrument used should be solid, not flexible, and should be large enough to cover a large portion of the skull region. The smaller the instrument, the smaller the surface area to be impacted and the greater the risk of pain to the animal. This technique should only be used in the most extreme of circumstances and when owners are not present.

### Electrocution

Electrocution is currently classified as an adjunctive method of euthanasia in dogs. To be considered euthanasia, dogs must be unconscious and completely unaware of the electrical current being passed through their body. What makes this technique objectionable is the violent physical activity demonstrated by the dog that the observer must bear witness to. Because other techniques are far superior, its training will not be listed here.

## Special circumstances

Scientific study shows that embryos and fetuses cannot experience pain and breathlessness during pregnancy and "cannot suffer while dying in utero after the death of the dam, whatever the cause" (Mellor 2010). Once their first breath is taken following birth, it is perceived that they experience pain and appropriate techniques should be utilized. Pregnant bitches and queens may be euthanized via IV or IC injection with death of the fetuses occurring naturally from anesthetic overdose or hypoxia soon afterward. This may take up to 15-20 minutes after the mother is confirmed dead (AVMA euthanasia guideline review 2011). IP injections of pentobarbital should be avoided during the later stages of pregnancy. The uterus may be accidentally injected and thus unable to be rapidly absorbed. However, IP injections are perfectly acceptable for the newborns as venous access can be very difficult. It may be necessary to euthanize fetuses still within the uterus during caesarian section of the pregnant bitch or queen. This can be safely accomplished by clamping the uterine blood vessels, thus allowing the fetuses to die by hypoxia.

Physical methods used on dogs and cats are only recommended when study requires it or no other options are available, especially with client-owned pets. These methods, such as blunt force trauma, can be very difficult to watch, let alone perform. It is recognized that technical challenges may arise during more preferred techniques and physical methods must then be used. Onlookers should be prepared for physical changes in the pet that will undoubtedly occur.

## Exotics

### Inhalant agents
#### *Ferrets*
Often, ferrets are presented in poor body condition, being emaciated and severely dehydrated. Each case must be evaluated considering the skill level of the handler, the condition of the animal, and the ability to discuss these issues with the owner. A very moribund ferret with marked dehydration, but normal respirations, can easily be sedated using a cotton ball soaked with isoflurane anesthesia liquid. Other gas anesthesia liquids that can be used are halothane, enflurane, sevoflurane, methoxyflurane, and desflurane. The soaked cotton ball is placed in an enclosed container such as a facemask used for the anesthesia machine or a plastic bag. Due to the corrosive nature of isoflurane in its liquid form, an old facemask used only for this purpose is recommended. It is important not to allow direct contact of the soaked cotton ball with the animal or the owner. The animal's head is placed in the mask or plastic bag with the rest of the body extending out the other end of the mask where the owner can stroke the pet if desired (Figure 5.19). It will generally take approximately 2–3 minutes for the sedation to render an unconscious state (no response to toe pinch and loss of palpebral reflex).

If the ferret is severely debilitated, this form of sedation will often cause respiratory arrest within less than a minute, and cardiac arrest usually occurs within approximately 1–3 minutes. It is recommended to inform the owner that further assistance may be needed such as an injectable euthanasia solution if the heart continues to beat.

Inhalation of an anesthetic gas is a very rapid and calm method for sedating and/or euthanizing a ferret. The owner is usually much calmer with this procedure because their pet does not have to be injected with a needle. Any struggling that may occur happens when the mask is applied; within one to two breaths an immediate calming and anesthesia is achieved. The struggle is usually very minor, especially if the ferret is in a very poor state of health. There may be a period of brief panic if the ferret is active, alert, and in relatively fair condition. In this author's experience, many owners still prefer this method rather than an injection.

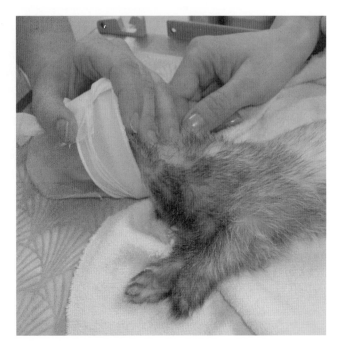

**Figure 5.19** A ferret in a face mask sealed at the end with an isoflurane-soaked cotton ball in the end of mask.

### Rabbits

The same method of an isoflurane-soaked cotton ball works well in very small, less than 2-lb rabbits or very debilitated rabbits. If they have severe respiratory disease, this method may take longer to be effective due to the decreased function of the respiratory tract. This method will sedate a small or debilitated rabbit with as few as three to four breaths or it may completely euthanize them. Within 2-3 minutes, euthanasia solution can be administered, if necessary, by IV, IP, or intraorgan injection.

### Guinea pigs, chinchillas, rats, hamsters, gerbils, mice, and sugar gliders

These animals generally do not tolerate handling without a tremendous amount of stress; therefore, any discomfort experienced from the odor of the gas anesthetic is much less than the stress experienced from handling. Therefore, the most humane and calm method for euthanizing these animals is using the isoflurane-soaked cotton ball in a mask. The mask can be held over the face or a larger mask can be placed over the entire animal, as for the small pocket pets or sugar gliders (Figure 5.20).

There may be a brief period of less than 20 seconds of mild struggling due to the animal's discontent of being confined and then they usually relax. Respiratory arrest occurs within 30-60 seconds and cardiac arrest occurs shortly thereafter, generally within another 5-20 seconds. If the owner wants to hold the animal, they can do so once the animal is anesthetized in the large

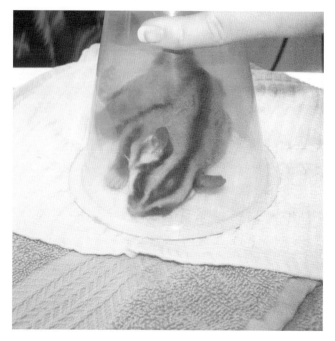

**Figure 5.20**  A sugar glider in a large facemask.

facemask and then the large facemask can be immediately replaced with a small facemask that fits over the animal's face. This mask needs to be readily available because the whole process occurs so rapidly that the animal may be euthanized before the small facemask is placed. Another option is to have the animal on a towel on the owner's lap with the large facemask over the entire animal for the whole procedure. Again, the client should be protected from touching or inhaling the isoflurane liquid by keeping the setup sealed as much as possible. To facilitate this, the masks used over the face of these small animals can have a latex glove taped over the large opening instead of the typical black rubber end. A smaller opening can be cut into the latex glove to keep the mask more airtight (Figure 5.21).

The isoflurane-soaked cotton ball is usually enough to euthanize the smaller animals, but in cases where it only anesthetizes the larger ones such as the guinea pigs, rabbits, or chinchillas, a euthanasia injectable agent can be administered IP, IC, or intraorgan. Generally, if the soaked cotton ball method is used, cardiac arrest should occur within 3–4 minutes. If it has not occurred within this time frame, then the euthanasia solution should be administered. The smaller and more sealed the container that the animal is placed in with the soaked cotton ball, the more rapid and effective the inhalant drug is.

There have been times when two of the family pets have needed euthanized at the same time such as two guinea pigs and they have been placed in a small plastic shoebox together. They were more comfortable together and the cotton ball method worked quite well. Both animals were calm and died very

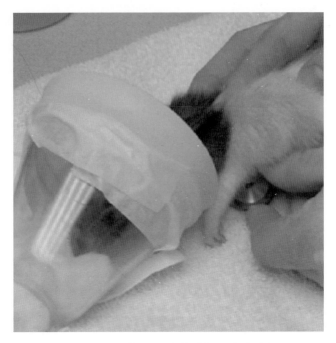

**Figure 5.21** A rat in a smaller facemask that is sealed with an isoflurane-soaked cotton ball at the end.

quietly. For highly fractious animals that are more dangerous to handle such as prairie dogs, skunks, squirrels, raccoons, or even the occasional ferret, a similar closed system can be devised using a plastic bag over a trap, squeeze cage, or small carrier and the gas anesthetic can be administered with several soaked isoflurane cotton balls or if available the gas anesthetic machine, though this method can take much longer.

$CO_2$ delivered by a $CO_2$ chamber (not dry ice) must be slowly delivered at a rate no higher than 5 psi or 1 L/min for a small cage or 4.5 L/min in a large cage (University of Minnesota, guidelines for euthanasia).

### Reptiles

Given the reptilian's slow metabolism and ability to hold their breath for long periods of time, euthanasia or anesthesia using inhalant gases is conditionally acceptable by the AVMA, but is not generally recommended. Many reptiles and amphibians are capable of breath holding and shunting of their blood, which permits conversion to anaerobic metabolism for survival during prolonged periods of anoxia; up to 27 hours for some species (AVMA euthanasia guideline review 2011). Because of this, induction of anesthesia and time to loss of consciousness may be greatly prolonged when inhalants are used. Studies by Burns (1995) and Baier (2006) have demonstrated that death may not occur even with prolonged exposure. Chelonians are more resistant to hypoxia than lizards and snakes, which lends them to being the least affected by gas anesthesia.

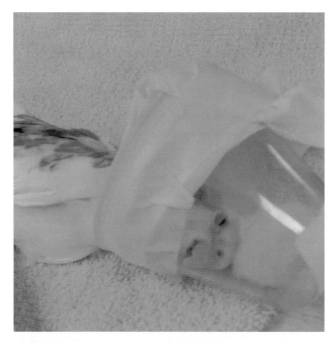

**Figure 5.22** Cockatiel in an enclosed facemask with a latex glove at the open end and an isofluorane-soaked cotton ball in the mask.

### Amphibians

Because amphibians can hold their breath similar to that of reptiles, inhalant anesthetics are not recommended for euthanasia. $CO_2$ is also an unacceptable method of euthanasia for amphibians due to their ability to survive for extended periods in a low oxygen environment (Brown 2003).

### Birds

Most birds weighing less than 500 g are easily and quickly euthanized using an anesthetic-soaked cotton ball. The choice of gas anesthesia used on the cotton ball can be one of several such as isoflurane, halothane, enflurane, and sevoflurane. The cotton ball is placed in a facemask, plastic bottle, or the long end of a syringe case with a latex glove on the open end to help seal it around the face (Figure 5.22). It can also be placed in the end of a small plastic bag that is rolled up enough to just cover the face, which works well when doing the procedure with the client present.

Any of these can be attempted with the client present. With some birds, there may be a brief moment of struggle as they inhale the anesthetic, but this quickly passes within just 1–3 breaths. Respiratory arrest occurs generally within 20–60 seconds depending on the size of the bird. Cardiac arrest generally occurs within 1–2 minutes after respiratory arrest. The heart must be monitored closely to determine time of death. The bird should be kept within the gas chamber setup during the confirmation of death as they may recover quickly if death has not been achieved.

For larger birds, the anesthetic-soaked cotton ball can be used to anesthetize them enough to then give the injection of euthanasia solution. Note that there may be a brief excitement stage of a few seconds, which can be quite disconcerting to the owner if they are not forewarned. The bird may also struggle if the handlers are not prepared with proper restraint techniques, especially when working with the larger geese, roosters, peafowl, and other large game birds. These birds have strong wings that can inflict harm to the handlers if they are not held firmly enough. It is generally recommended to use injectable sedation or anesthetic drugs for these large birds for the handler's safety and the bird's comfort.

### Fish

Inhalant drugs such as isoflurane and halothane can be distributed into the water bath for inhalation across the gills. This is often done with oxygen, but the levels are unreliable due to the insoluble nature of the drugs. For fish too large for immersion, the anesthetic water can be poured over the gills directly. $CO_2$ and CO have been frequently used as euthanasia agents, but again it is difficult to maintain an accurate level of concentration in the water and a high level of oxygen must be administered as well. (Neiffer and Stamper 2009). Since $CO_2$ is the only chemical without tissue residues, the fish may become part of the food chain such as fishmeal or food for human consumption (University of Florida IFAS Extension).

### Technical challenges

As mentioned previously, there are numerous challenges that present when working with inhalant gases. The first is the inherent risk of gas leaking from the chamber itself. When clients are present, every caution must be taken to seal the contraption as much as possible, especially in the presence of a pregnant woman as these gases can pose health risks to the fetus. Clients should be alerted that inhalant gases have odors and if they smell them, they need to notify the veterinarian and staff immediately. Leaking gas also slows the time of anesthesia induction and death because less is readily available for the pet to inhale.

Anesthetic gases all have odors associated with them, which may make for brief struggling as described. Each animal must be properly restrained to avoid injury to themselves and the handler. If this is deemed too difficult, an injectable sedative or anesthetic can be given quickly and the animal released back into its home cage to prevent added stress. The animal can then relax in its own space and be removed for euthanasia when ready. If the animal refuses to breathe due to the odor, there is little that can be done to stimulate inhalation, especially with regard to reptiles and amphibians.

In the presence of respiratory disease, the animal may be unable to rapidly absorb the drugs across the alveolar surface. This will lengthen the time to anesthesia or death. Families should be warned that the process may take longer than normal. If deemed necessary, a second method should be utilized.

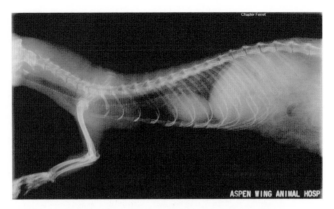

**Figure 5.23**  Radiograph of a ferret showing the heart location.

## Noninhalant pharmaceutical agents
### Injectable methods
Most exotics can be euthanized via a variety of injectable methods using barbiturates and barbiturate-combination drugs. They may also be given overdoses of injectable anesthetics similar to dogs and cats. The following represents those injectable techniques that are easily accomplished in private practice with or without owners present.

### Ferret
If venous access is possible, cephalic or lateral saphenous veins can be used. The cephalic vein is located on the dorsal surface of the front limb as in the dog, and the lateral saphenous vein is located laterally on the hind limb above the hock joint. If the euthanasia solution being used is thick, diluting the solution 50/50 with saline, so it will flow more easily through a 25-gauge needle, works well. Generally, it is advisable to be generous with the solution if in front of the owner. Even though only 1 mL may be required for an IV barbiturate injection, using 4-6 cc total of the diluted solution is not uncommon.

If venous access is impossible, an IC injection can be performed on an anesthetized animal using a 22-gauge 1-in. needle. Note that the ferret's heart is located more caudally than other domestic pets, between the 7th and 10th ICS (Figure 5.23). The needle should be directed perpendicular to the heart, similar to that done in cats and dogs.

The euthanasia solution can also be delivered IP using 2 cc of full strength solution. This method may take up to 10-15 minutes due to the rate of natural absorption across membranes. Other routes of administering euthanasia solution include intrahepatic, especially if there is hepatomegaly present, or intrarenal; however, this can be difficult in an overweight ferret or one with a large amount of ascites. Also, one must consider the large amount of perirenal fat normally present in ferrets. Again, these methods of injections must be done in an anesthetized animal.

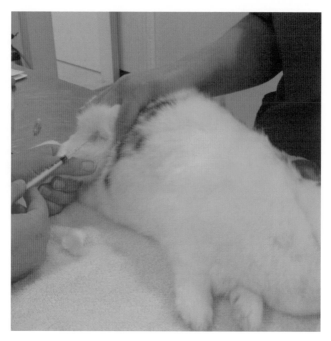

**Figure 5.24** Accessing the medial, saphenous vein in a rabbit.

### Rabbits

The venous sights include cephalic, lateral saphenous, marginal ear veins, and jugular veins. The jugular vein can be very difficult to access and can be very stressful for the awake rabbit when forced to lay in an unnatural position. The marginal ear veins are preferred in an awake rabbit due to the low stress involved for handling the rabbit for this venous access.

If the rabbit is hydrated, all veins are usually large enough to pass a 25-gauge needle into. Following the ear vein, the medial, saphenous vein is the next choice of vein and is located on the lateral region of the tibia (Figure 5.24). Shaving the fur is not necessary and can be stressful to the rabbit. In the awake rabbit, it should be held snuggly in a towel and slightly tilted on its side. This vein can easily be located using a small amount of alcohol on a cotton ball to part the hair to visualize the vein. Rabbits do not tolerate a lateral position well, so keeping them just slightly tilted decreases anxiety. The handler can hold the hind leg firmly, gripping the proximal one-third of the leg so the vein is held off.

The cephalic vein can also be used. It is preferred for use in an anesthetized or sedated rabbit as they generally do not tolerate their front legs being handled. In general, if the euthanasia fluid is to be administered by the IV route, it may be preferred that the rabbit be sedated prior to the IV injection to decrease stress. Euthanasia solution should be diluted 50/50 if it is thick, as was described for the ferret, and given slowly.

Nondebilitated rabbits tend to have a large amount of abdominal fat, and a peritoneal injection of euthanasia fluid can take a very long time to be

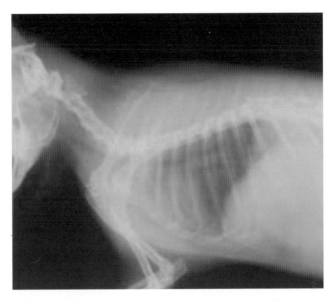

**Figure 5.25** Radiograph of a rabbit showing the heart location.

absorbed. In rabbits with hepatomegaly, the liver may be the preferred intraorgan injection. Kidneys can be difficult to access whether the rabbit is debilitated or in good flesh due to the normally large amount of abdominal and perirenal fat present in most rabbits. For IC injections, note that the heart in rabbits is located more cranial between the 1st and 5th ICS (Figure 5.25).

### Guinea pigs, chinchillas, rats, hamsters, gerbils, mice, and sugar gliders
IV injection in these pocket pets is very challenging and often avoided by veterinarians, especially when owners are present. The time and effort to find a usable vein can create stress for those watching. Other routes of injectable administration are preferred. IC administration in the small pocket pets may be quite challenging or intimidating to some people, so other organs can be used.

### Reptiles
Reasons to euthanize reptiles are similar to that of other species of animals and should be done in a humane manner. Injection of a noninhalant pharmaceutical agent such as a barbiturate or barbiturate-combination drug is the most common technique used in reptiles in private practice. They do not readily accept inhalant gases and the physical methods commonly used in other species do not work well with their unique anatomy; however, these other methods may be used in certain circumstances when injectable agents are unavailable. The method of euthanasia is important to consider if a necropsy or histopathology will be desired.

As discussed in a previous section, reptiles may be given pre-euthanasia sedation/anesthesia to facilitate safer handling and less pain during euthanasia itself. A few techniques listed in the following text do not require

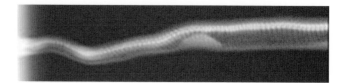

**Figure 5.26** Radiograph of a snake with the head to the left and the opacity in the center is the heart, which on this snake is approximately 1/4 distal from the head.

anesthesia for them to be acceptable, however, it may be necessary to guarantee a smooth euthanasia, especially for those unfamiliar with the species.

It can be very difficult to assess if a reptile patient is dead or alive especially, when it is very cold. They also do not metabolize the drugs well when cold, therefore, slowing the process down significantly. It is absolutely necessary to assure that the animal is truly dead and keeping the body 24 hours prior to sending it home with the client may be advisable. There have been cases where the euthanized reptile was found walking around in the plastic bag the next day. Additionally, those animals whose bodies will be taken home with the client, should be given at least three times the recommended volume of euthanasia drug (Mader 1996).

### Assessing the heartbeat in reptiles

In snakes, it helps to make a discrete mark with a marker pen at the location of the heart so it will be easier to find once the animal is sedated or anesthetized. The heartbeat can generally be seen through the scales or a doplar can be used to locate the heart. The general location of the heart in the snake is 1/4-1/3 distal from the head. For chelonians (turtles and tortoises), the doplar probe can be placed in the front area between the neck and forelimb so the heartbeat can be monitored throughout the process, as it can be very difficult to assess the occurrence of death in these animals (see Figures 5.26-5.29).

### Lizards

Lizards are commonly euthanized by injecting either the ventral tail vein or the ventral abdominal vein. For ventral tail injections, the lizard can be restrained by wrapping it firmly in a towel in dorsal or sternal recumbency leaving the ventral tail area open for venipuncture. The dorsal position is easier to work with in a sedated lizard, while the sternal position is less stressful for an awake lizard. A 25-22-gauge needle on syringe is inserted perpendicularly to the tail between the scales, midline, and approximately 1/3-1/2 distal distance from the cloaca to the tip of the tail. The needle must reach the vertebral column so it is helpful to measure the thickness of the tail at the location where the needle will be inserted. The needle is inserted perpendicular to the tail until the caudal vertebrae is contacted. The veterinarian will then apply gentle negative pressure on the syringe while carefully and slowly withdrawing the needle until blood flow is achieved. The euthanasia solution is then administered. In the sternal position, the lizard can be supported by a table and the tail draped over

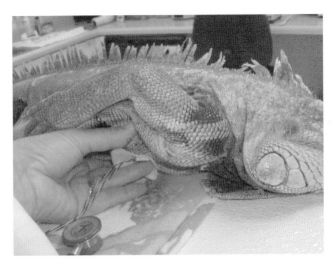

**Figure 5.27** Doplar location in a lizard.

the edge, making sure the tail is held firmly to prevent injury to the handler and the lizard (Figure 5.30).

For access to the ventral abdominal vein, the lizard should be sedated or anesthetized to render it motionless. In this author's experience, this vein is easy to tear and can bleed excessively. The lizard should be placed in dorsal recumbency. Using a 22–25-gauge needle, the vein, located just under the skin, is accessed by inserting the needle midline between the umbilical scar and the cloaca (Figure 5.31).

For performing IC injections, the heart can be found in the cranial coelomic cavity and is accessed through the thoracic inlet. Veterinarians will need to insert a 0.5–2-in., 22–25-gauge needle into the thoracic inlet just above the symphysis of the clavicles (Figure 5.32). The needle is directed caudally and

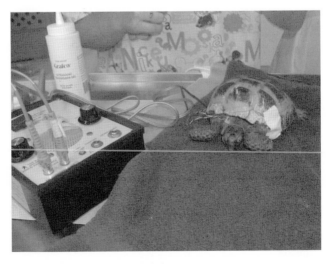

**Figure 5.28** Doplar setup for a tortoise.

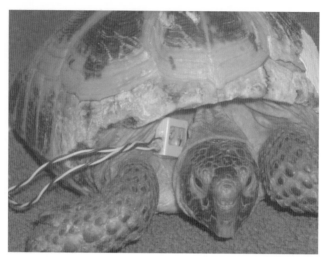

**Figure 5.29** Doplar location for a tortoise.

parallel to the base of the sternum, applying gentle negative pressure while advancing until blood enters the syringe.

### Snakes

Snakes differ from lizards in that the ventral abdominal vein is rarely ever used. The ventral caudal tail vein is preferred and is accessed using a 25-22-gauge needle, between 5/8 and 1 in. in length. The needle is inserted between scales, approximately one-third the distance caudal to the cloaca between the cloaca and tip of tail in a craniodorsal angle. The veterinarian will apply gentle negative pressure in the syringe once the needle is through the skin until the

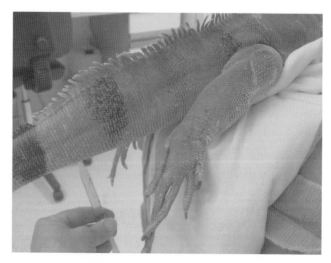

**Figure 5.30** Intravenous (IV) injection into the ventral caudal tail vein of an iguana.

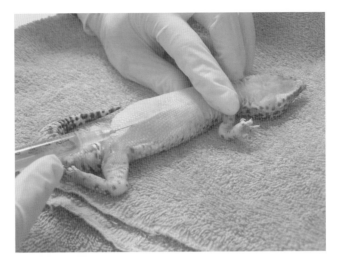

**Figure 5.31** Ventral abdominal vein access in a leopard gecko.

vessel is located (Figure 5.33). It is close to the level of the vertebrae as in the lizard.

The heart location is variable with the species of snake, which can make IC injections more challenging, especially for those veterinarians unfamiliar with them. The heart can be visualized with the snake in dorsal recumbency and by watching for movement of the scutes, the large scales on the ventral surface. It can be stabilized using a thumb and finger at the heart's cranial

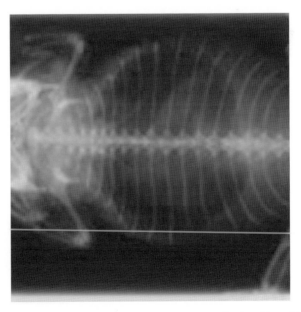

**Figure 5.32** Radiograph of a bearded dragon. Note the location of the heart is in the cranial aspect of the coelomic cavity.

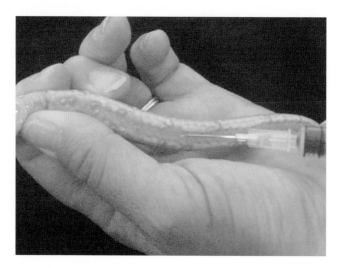

**Figure 5.33**  Ventral caudal tail vein insertion; note the cloaca at thumb.

and caudal position. A 0.5-2-in., 21-25-gauge needle can then be advanced perpendicularly into the heart to the suspected depth.

### Chelonians

Because of the thickness of their scales and the short length of their legs and tail, IV injections are rarely attempted in turtles and tortoises. In small chelonians, with the chelonian in sternal recumbency, a 1.5-2-in. 21-25-gauge needle is inserted into the thoracic inlet area and using gentle negative pressure, the needle is advanced until blood enters the syringe (Figure 5.34). The heart is injected while unconscious, similar to other species.

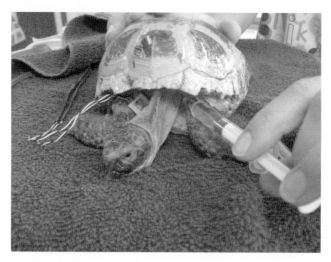

**Figure 5.34**  Intracardiac (IC) injection in a chelonian; note the doplar on the right side of the thoracic inlet monitoring the heart while injecting.

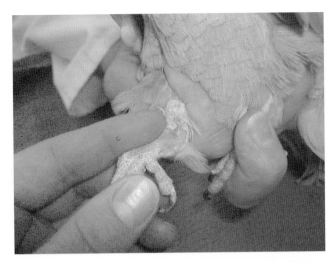

**Figure 5.35** The medial metatarsal vein can be seen on this amazon parrot.

### Amphibians

Barbiturates such as sodium pentobarbital can be given IV at a dose of 100 mg/kg when possible or a weaker concentration of 60 mg/ml can be given intracoelomic (ICo). MS-222 is another drug that can be injected ICo at a dose of 200 mg/kg (Brown 2003).

### Birds

For IV administration, the vein that would be most accessible is the leg vein, called the medial metatarsal vein, on the medial surface of the leg just proximal to the scaled portion of the foot. This is a common and easily accessible vein to obtain in large birds such as the ducks, chickens, game birds, and raptors, but can be used in some smaller species. The bird is wrapped in a towel and the handler stabilizes the leg at the stifle. The veterinarian then holds the foot firmly to inject the euthanasia solution (Figures 5.35 and 5.36). The smallest needle size should be chosen due to the small and fragile nature of this vein.

The wing vein (ulnar or brachial vein) as it crosses over the medial surface of the elbow joint can be easily accessed in larger birds. The bird is wrapped in a towel and the wing is gently pulled out away from the body (Figure 5.37). It is helpful to dampen the feathers at the medial surface of the elbow to visualize the vein.

The jugular vein is another venous access point, which is located on the right side of the neck in the featherless tract. Birds have a jugular vein on either side, but the right jugular vein is larger, and therefore, easier to inject. The jugular vein is more difficult to access in columbiformes, such as pigeons and doves, as there is no lateral cervical apterium (featherless tract). These birds also have a diffuse venous plexus rather than a single jugular vein.

To access the jugular vein, the bird is wrapped in a towel and the right side of the neck is exposed by gently stretching the neck. The handler must hold

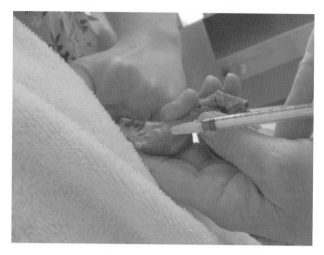

**Figure 5.36** The bird is wrapped in a towel and the handler is stabilizing the leg while the clinician is holding the foot firmly and injecting into the medial metatarsal vein.

the head and beak firmly with their right hand and control the body with their left hand, taking care not to apply pressure over the keel bone (breast bone). Birds do not have diaphragms. They control their breathing by moving their keel bone up and down, so any firm pressure on the keel will result in distress and hypoxia (Figure 5.38).

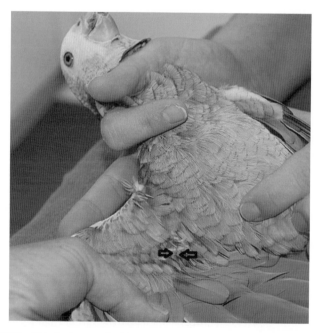

**Figure 5.37** This is demonstrating the position of the bird without the towel to utilize the ulnar or wing vein.

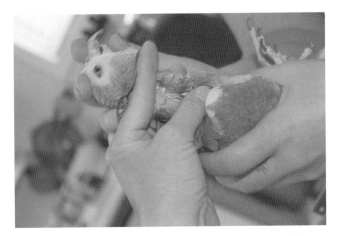

**Figure 5.38** The larger, more accessible jugular vein is located on the right side of the neck in the featherless tract. The position of the bird and head are shown here.

When venous access is impossible, an intrahepatic, IC, or ICo injection can be given with the bird in a state of unconsciousness. The intrahepatic injection will only be possible if there is hepatomegaly due to the presence of the long breastbone impeding the injection site. ICo injections can be done easily, but may take a longer period of time to be absorbed. IC injections can be performed using a 1.5–2-in., 22-gauge needle and angling the needle down caudally into the thoracic inlet. Once there, the veterinarian must aspirate with the syringe deep enough, and when the heart is penetrated, visualize blood flow before injecting the solution (Figures 5.39 and 5.40).

*Fish*
Sodium pentobarbital may be injected at a dose of 100 mg/kg given IV or ICo, or given at 0.22 mL/kg IV or ICo (UMN 2009). Some injectables are acceptable in fish. Pentobarbital by itself is perfectly acceptable. If the fish requires

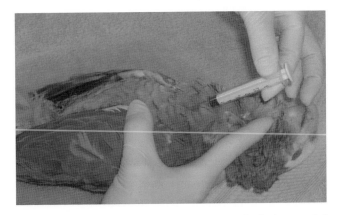

**Figure 5.39** Intracardiac (IC) injection with the needle facing caudally down into the thoracic inlet.

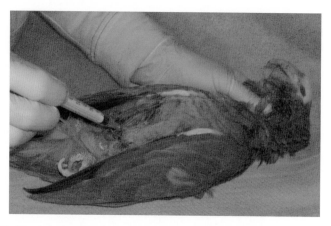

**Figure 5.40** Intrahepatic injection with the needle under the distal point of the keel bone facing cranially.

pre-euthanasia anesthesia, ketamine or a combination of ketamine and medetomidine, and propofol are acceptable drugs to give, followed by pentobarbital (AVMA euthanasia guideline review 2011). Ketamine can lead to muscle spasms during induction, so the client should be aware of this. Anesthesia followed by IV KCl at 1-2 meq/kg is an acceptable method. (University of Minnesota guidelines)

### Immersion and topical methods

#### Amphibians

Amphibians have a unique characteristic to their anatomy that allows for another method of euthanasia. The amphibian's skin is highly permeable and will absorb drugs quite readily. Some amphibians also have secretions on their skin that can be harmful or even quite toxic to our skin; therefore, it is always advisable to handle them with gloves. It is also much less irritating to the amphibian's skin if the gloves are rinsed with distilled water to wash off any talc powder (Mader 1996).

The amphibian is placed in a shallow bath of only a few millimeters of the liquid drug and the drug will be absorbed through the ventral surface of the skin (Figure 5.41). As with any procedure, care must be taken to ensure that the animal is dead, using a stethoscope to monitor heart rate as well as monitoring respirations. If necessary, pithing or freezing can be done once the animal is completely anesthetized or administering an injection of commercial euthanasia drug at 0.22 mL/kg or an overdose of barbiturate at 100-200 mg/kg ICo or IC.

The following drugs for the bath can be used:

- *Ethyl alcohol bath*: The animal is placed in a 5% solution until anesthetized, at which time it can be moved to a stronger solution or another technique utilized for more rapid results.
- *MS-222*: A 0.3% (3 g/L) solution is effective in most species of amphibians to cause deep anesthesia within just a few minutes. Cardiac arrest by this

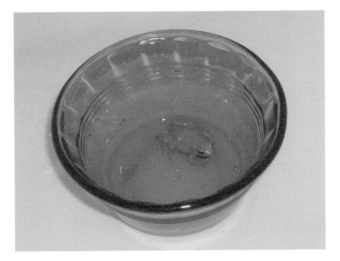

**Figure 5.41** Frog in shallow bath of MS-222.

method alone may take up to 5 hours. An injection of euthanasia solution may be needed to assist the time of death. MS-222 is acidic at >500 mg/L and must be buffered to a pH of 7.0-7.5. This can be done using sodium bicarbonate at 2 g per g of MS-222.

- *Benzocaine HCl–Orajel®*: The effects of this chemical are similar to MS-222. It is also very acidic and needs to be neutralized to a pH of 7.0-7.5 using sodium bicarbonate. Benzocaine HCl is also available over the counter in forms such as Orajel of which the 7.5% and 20% are both effective. The chemical is easy to obtain and effective to use.

One reference describes the Orajel being placed directly on the ventral abdomen of the amphibian and the animal is then placed in a plastic bag. This method is very rapid, usually taking effect in less than a minute and seems to work best in anurans (frogs, toads). A 5-mm drop placed on the ventral abdomen will result in rapid death of a dwarf salamander (Brown 2003; Torreilles et al. 2009).

Note that straight benzocaine is not water-soluble, and therefore, not recommended; benzocaine HCl must be used to be effective.


### Fish

For obvious reasons, immersion and dermal absorption is the euthanasia method of choice for fish. The use of MS-222 using a solution of 2 g/L of water is recommended. This technique may take from 20 minutes up to 3 hours to achieve death, and therefore, a physical method may need to be used once unconsciousness is obtained. The pH must be adjusted to 7 using sodium bicarbonate. Another immersion solution is benzocaine HCl (Orajel) at 250 mg/L of water. Magnesium sulfate/magnesium chloride may also be used in a water bath. Fish should be left in the solution for a minimum of 10 minutes after cessation of opercular movement (AVMA euthanasia guideline review 2011).

### Technical challenges

Exotics euthanized with noninhalant pharmaceutical agents tend to pose challenges simply due to their unique anatomy. IV injections are considered more difficult in most exotics due to small vein size, the presence of scales and feathers, etc. When venous access cannot be found, or stress to an awake animal is considered too great, IP injections with a barbiturate may be performed in small mammals.

ICo injections in reptiles are not recommended due to the prolonged time involved compared with the time it takes to complete euthanasia via the IV or IC route in an anesthetized animal. Additionally, injecting chloroform is no longer recommended due to the pain this drug causes (McCarthur et al. 2004, Mader 1996).

## Physical methods

### Cervical dislocation

*Mice, rats, small rabbits and birds, reptiles* Cervical dislocation may be necessary in situations where there is no equipment available or as secondary means of assuring death after injectable euthanasia and should only be done by trained personnel. This should only be done in animals less than 0.5 kg and the animal should be sedated or unconscious. The AVMA lists turkeys as an acceptable species for this technique as well. The animal should be heavily sedated or anesthetized whenever possible, especially if the veterinarian is new to the technique. A small board, dowel, or pencil (depending on the size of animal) can be placed at the base of the animal's skull. With a rapid strong pull at the base of the tail, the veterinarian will simultaneously push down firmly against the board to separate the first cervical from the skull. The board placed at the base of the skull helps stabilize the head. Veterinarians and others attempting this with their fingers will tend to hesitate as they feel a definite crunching of bones. Using a board or rod minimizes the risk of incomplete dislocation of the cervical vertebrae (Figure 5.42).

There will often be a large amount of postmortem thrashing. Again, verification that respiratory and cardiac arrest has occurred is crucial. Because this technique is technically difficult, proper training, including practicing on deceased pocket pets first, may be helpful. The AVMA classifies it as conditionally acceptable on small pocket pets and turkeys. A fair amount of force on mammals larger than rats is needed, and therefore, it is not recommended when other techniques are available. For obvious reasons, this method should not be done in front of a client.

### Birds

Cervical dislocation is accomplished using a board or small dowel and is done using the same technique as in the mammals and reptiles. Firm downward pressure is applied on the board with a quick strong pull of the body. The head of the smaller birds is often popped off with this method due to the force applied and there is a crunching of bone beneath the board. There is often dramatic postmortem thrashing with this technique. This method can

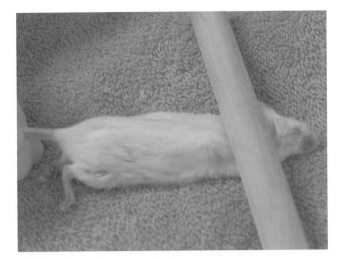

**Figure 5.42** Cervical dislocation of a rat.

be used on the larger water fowl and game birds such as geese and pheasants by grasping the base of the head with one hand and the base of the neck with the other and pulling rapidly and firmly in opposite directions with a snapping action (Figures 5.43 and 5.44). Once again, this should be done in an anesthetized bird.

### Technical challenges
There will be times when it is physically impossible for the veterinarian to achieve proper cervical dislocation. Whether the neck is too thick or the veterinarian lacks the strength to break the neck, another method will have to be

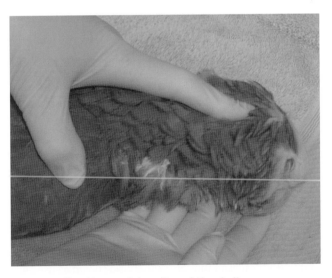

**Figure 5.43** Locating the caudal portion of the skull.

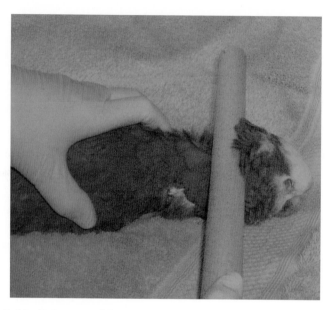

**Figure 5.44** Using a small board just caudal to the skull and a hand is placed on the body for cervical dislocation.

rapidly employed. This is never ideal and can cause stress to the veterinarian and observers. If a rod or board is not available, anything can be used to hold the head in place such as the edge of a book, stapler, etc. The more awkward the object to hold, the greater the risk of improper technique.

### Gunshot and captive bolt

Pet crocodilians and other large reptiles can be euthanized by a penetrating captive bolt or gunshot (free bullet) delivered to the brain. The gun should be aimed at the brain, which would be along the midsagittal plane and just caudal to the eyes (Mader 1996).

### Decapitation

*Small mammals, reptiles, amphibians, birds, fish* Decapitation can be used as a sole method of euthanasia or as an adjunctive method to guarantee death following another method. It is an option in smaller reptiles and should be done in an anesthetized animal. The force and positioning of the strike to the skull has to be strong enough and very accurate to cause rapid death. A sharp instrument such as a guillotine blade or other sharp blade such as an osteotome would suffice, taking care to avoid personnel injury. This is a rapid way to kill a reptile but the brain must be destroyed for it to be a humane method, as the brain in reptiles can stay viable for up to an hour (Cooper et al. 1984; Kaplans 1994).

Decapitation can be done on amphibians and then should be followed with pithing. Physical methods of euthanasia should be used in an anesthetized bird and include decapitation and cervical dislocation. Decapitation can be done

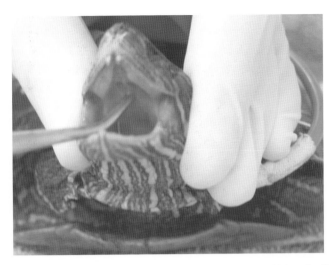

**Figure 5.45** Pithing the brain through the roof of the mouth in a turtle.

with a sharp blade or shears in the small birds as the finches. The blade is placed just caudal to the skull to separate the skull from the first vertebrae.

### Freezing

There have been various methods of euthanasia used in the past that would not be considered humane with current standards. One such method is placing the animal in a freezer to lower the body temperature enough to cause death. This method is very painful in that the freezing causes ice crystals to form in the tissues. If such a method is used, it should be in an anesthetized animal only (Kaplans 1994; Mader 1996).

### Pithing

Pithing the brain and spinal cord or crushing the skull over or just caudal to the region over the eyes is a common adjunctive technique in exotic animals. Pithing the brain can be done with a sharp dental probe inserted through the foramen magnum with the spike rotated to destroy the brain tissue. Another method of pithing can be done by inserting the dental probe through the roof of the mouth into the cranial vault. The spike is then rotated to destroy the brain tissue (Figures 5.45 and 5.46). The latter method may be preferred for animals being sent home after euthanasia (McCarthur 2004). For obvious reasons, these methods should not be done in front of the client. Pithing and decapitation would be the methods used to be sure death has occurred.

### Special circumstances

Many exotic species lay eggs as their form of reproduction. Eggs with embryos may be destroyed by prolonged exposure (20 minutes) to $CO_2$, cooling (4 hours

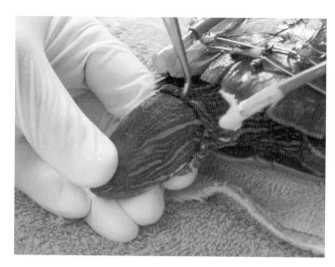

**Figure 5.46** Pithing the brain through the foramen magnum using a dental probe.

at 40 °F), or freezing (Close 1997). In some cases inhalant anesthetics can be administered through the air cell at the large end of the egg. Egg addling can also be used (Orosz 2006).

Little information is available on the sensory capacity of amphibians and reptiles at the egg stage of development (Close 1997). Fresh oviposited eggs may be euthanized using rapid freezing or maceration, both of which result in instantaneous death. More developed eggs should be euthanized like adults since little is known about the physiology of life inside.

Exotics with altricial young, such as mice and rats, must be differentiated from those with precocial young, such as guinea pigs. Precocial young should be treated as adults. In utero, like many other species, the fetuses are not believed to experience pain and breathlessness due to the death of the dam (Mellor et al. 2005). Fetuses may be euthanized in the same manner as adults, but as described before, young animals tend to be more resistant to hypoxia, and therefore, inhalants should be avoided if possible. Inhalants are classified as conditionally acceptable in neonates. Neonatal mice may take up to 50 minutes to die from $CO_2$ exposure (Pritchett 2005). A secondary method may be needed. The AVMA does list hypothermia, the gradual cooling of fetuses/neonates, as a conditionally acceptable technique provided the animals do not directly contact ice (wet or dry) or precooled surfaces. This is not recommended after 7 days of age. Fetuses/neonates can be efficiently killed by rapidly freezing in liquid nitrogen, but they should be rendered unconscious first to be safe. Decapitation is also conditionally acceptable for altricial neonates younger than 5 days of age (AVMA euthanasia guideline review 2011). Once animals acquire hair, another method should be chosen.

Fish can undergo blunt force trauma, decapitation, freezing, and pithing like other species as long as unconsciousness and death are immediate.

## Horses

The actual process of euthanizing a horse, donkey, or mule needs to be orchestrated with safety for the people and humane treatment for the patient as the top two priorities. The patient needs to be moved away from other animals as they may present a distraction for the veterinarian and horse itself. Distractions often translate into safety issues. The owner may request to hold the horse, but profound grief may make them less effective at restraint and less responsive in keeping themselves safe. It is preferable to have a trained technician restrain the animal. In some cases, especially when using a firearm, the procedure may be performed without any assistance to minimize risk for those involved. Restraints such as stocks are rarely used due to the difficulty of extricating the body afterward. Any confined space including stalls or horse trailers increase the risk for the people involved because the avenues for escape are limited. It is important to emphasize to all involved that the horse's response to euthanasia, particularly barbiturate administration, may be unpredictable. They may sink quietly to the ground but may also fall over backward or lunge forward putting even an experienced horse handler at risk. When euthanizing a horse that is to be buried, it is often expedient to have the horse as close to the burial site as possible. This does add one more danger to the procedure. If the horse bolts or falls unexpectedly, the veterinarian may be pushed into the hole. It is even possible the horse could fall on top of the person. If the horse does fall directly into the hole, the attending veterinarian will have to climb in to verify death. Public events or horses requiring euthanasia in public settings add several complications. Often, the public wants to help the poor horse and while this is noble, it is misguided. Too many people in the area greatly increase the risk of someone getting hurt. An equine public event should have a team designated for such an emergency situation. It is optimum to get the horse out of the public view if humanely possible. A mechanism to remove the animal after euthanasia is also essential.

### Inhalant agents

The use of inhalant drugs to euthanize horses is rarely, if ever, attempted due to the availability of superior methods.

### Noninhalant pharmaceutical agents
#### Intravenous injections

The jugular vein is the most common site for IV injection of a euthanasia agent like pentobarbital. A catheter may be placed within the vein or direct venipuncture may be attempted. A local anesthetic or mild sedation may facilitate this process. Sedation can be useful for restraint during euthanasia, but the depressant effect on circulation may increase the time to loss of consciousness for the animal (AVMA euthanasia guideline review 2011). It is good to warn the client that there may also be increased muscular activity and agonal gasping when euthanizing a sedated horse. Sedation should still be used for excited or untrained horses or for horses in severe pain as from colic.

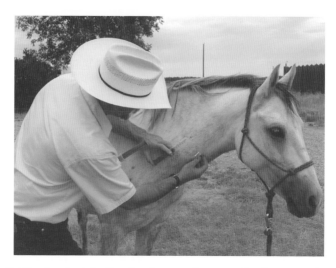

**Figure 5.47**   Jugular injection in a horse using a small extension set.

Once the injection site has been identified and prepared, the euthanasia procedure may be performed (Figures 5.47 and 5.48). The client should be consulted to be sure they are ready and the attending veterinarian and staff should survey the area one last time to be sure everyone is in safe positions. This means that onlookers and other animals are at least 20 ft away if possible.

Because euthanasia requires a large volume of drug, veterinarians will need to change syringes in the middle of the procedure. A second (and possibly third) syringe full of barbiturate should be readily available in a pocket or an experienced assistant may hand it to over when needed. The barbiturate

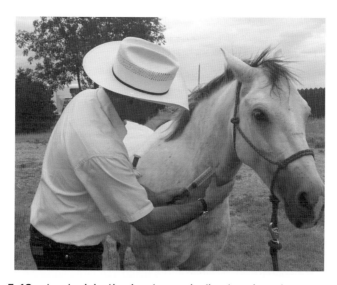

**Figure 5.48**   Jugular injection in a horse via direct venipuncture.

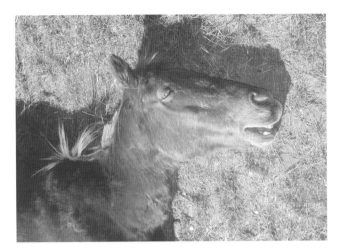

**Figure 5.49** A confirmed dead horse following barbiturate injection. Note the open eyes.

must be administered at a rapid rate. When the first syringe is empty, it may be discarded and quickly replaced with the second syringe. Some horses will drop before the first syringe of barbiturate is given. Others will still stand for several seconds after the full dose has been administered. Many horses will take a deep breath, then lose consciousness and fall. If the solution is administered too slowly, the horse may stumble a bit and appear anxious. This is never ideal for the client or veterinarian. A small amount of blood will leak from the injection site once the needle or catheter is removed.

Many veterinarians and assistants will be tempted to try and influence the way the animal falls to make it more esthetically acceptable to the owner. Pressure on the halter rope may prevent the head from hitting the ground, but can be difficult and possibly dangerous to those around. Understanding horse behavior and personal physical limitations will help prevent accidents.

The horse must be monitored for several minutes after it is down. Brain function will be inhibited by barbiturate anesthesia, but cardiac function may continue for several minutes. Additional doses of barbiturate may be needed if cardiac and respiratory functions continue. This author has seen animals with compromised circulatory systems that have required up to three times the expected dose of barbiturate to be effective. There are many sad stories of veterinarians that euthanized a horse with inadequate dose of drug and the horse "returned to life" several hours later. The patient's death must be verified using the corneal reflex, respiratory rate, and cardiac rate until all signs of life are absent (Figure 5.49).

### Technical challenges

Horses may have unpredictable reactions to barbiturate-induced euthanasia. They may stand for longer than expected, flip over backward, fall various directions, etc. If the horse has not become recumbent within a couple of minutes of barbiturate injection, more drug should be administered. Fifty to hundred percent of the first dose is usually an effective second dose.

Even in the most extreme of circumstances, a veterinarian should not allow themselves to run out of solution. If it did happen, due to poor planning or the horse's condition required more solution than expected, one must resort to another method. KCI administration would be appropriate if the horse is already unconscious, perhaps a physical method such as exsanguination or even gunshot would be appropriate.

In cases where the horse refuses to stand still for euthanasia, sedation will be required. If none is available, the veterinarian may have to consider aborting any attempt at a successful euthanasia. It is better than creating a disaster or getting injured.

If the jugular vein cannot be accessed for any reason, any vein that can be isolated is appropriate. The jugular is almost always accessible though and big in every horse. Trying to use a leg vein on a standing horse is never advised. If venous pressures are poor and the veins are difficult to feel, such as with a sick foal, an IC injection can be performed on unconscious animals using a large bore 4-6-in. needle.

## Physical methods
### Gunshot

When euthanasia is to be performed using a gunshot, safety must become the primary concern. The person using the firearm should have thorough knowledge of the gun being used and optimally would have completed a firearms safety course. All unnecessary personnel and other animals need to be away from the area. The report of the firearm and the animal dropping suddenly to the ground may be startling for people and for other animals. The client should be made aware that there will be bleeding from the bullet entry wound and from the nostrils.

Directing the path of the bullet in the animal is critical for a quick humane euthanasia. Clients that have attempted to euthanize their own horse using their personal firearm have quickly learned that proper placement is critical. They often find that after two to three firings, their horse is still standing. Education is the key to success with any technique, but improperly placed gunshots will be very stressing for everyone and obviously painful for the patient.

When the horse is in hand and a pistol is used, drawing the imaginary "X" on the forehead gives the best target. Attention to several details can dramatically increase the safety and efficacy of this technique. To begin, the veterinarian may hold the lead rope in one hand and the pistol in the other. This eliminates the need for an animal handler being placed in a potentially dangerous position. It is also much safer than tying the horse to something. The force of the horse going down may tear pieces from whatever it is tied to, which could injure onlookers. When positioning the gun, the barrel should not touch the horse. This may trigger the horse to move its head as the gun is fired, potentially disrupting the penetration point. The barrel of the pistol

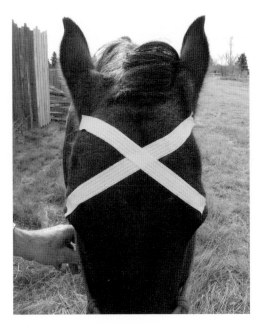

**Figure 5.50**  Frontal brain target in horses.

should be within 1-2 in. of the skin on the forehead. When the animal is facing the shooter, the target is the intersection of lines drawn from the base of the ear to the center of the eye on the opposite side (Figure 5.50; Wright 2009; CDFA 2010).

Another critically important point is to allow time for the horse to lower its head. If the shot is taken with the head elevated, the barrel of the gun will be level or pointed up (Figure 5.51).This may allow the bullet to deflect over the brain and exit the back of the skull. The barrel of the gun must be aligned with the horse's neck as shown in the picture (Figure 5.52).

The bullet will ideally travel through the brain and brain stem causing immediate unconsciousness and death. The bullet will remain in the neck decreasing risk to other animals or humans in the area. Sedation may be used to lower the head, but patience is all that is usually required to achieve this positioning. The veterinarian should wait until the horse lowers its head so the bullet will travel into the neck instead of exiting the back of the head. When veterinarians raise their hand with the pistol, most horses will raise their head. It is best to leave the gun elevated and reassure the horse. Almost all horses will bring their heads down in a few seconds allowing for proper alignment of the gun barrel and neck.

If the horse cannot be closely handled, such as in the case of an aggressive or frightened horse, a rifle can be used to place a bullet at the base of the ear from a lateral viewpoint (Figure 5.53).

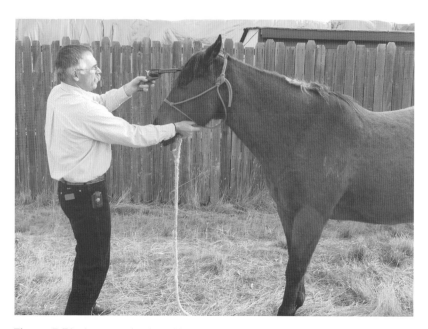

**Figure 5.51** Improperly placed frontal gunshot in a horse.

This will effectively disrupt brain and brainstem, but the bullet may exit the other side of the head. Obviously for safety reasons, this technique may only be used in limited circumstances. Shooting a horse in the neck or chest does not cause immediate loss of consciousness and is thus not acceptable by AVMA Guidelines on Euthanasia.

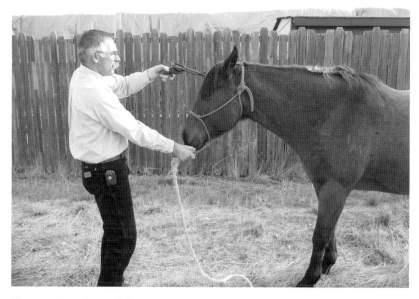

**Figure 5.52** Correct frontal gunshot placement in a horse.

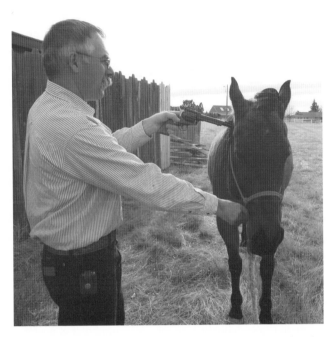

**Figure 5.53**   Ideal placement of a lateral gunshot to a horse's head.

### Technical challenges

Physical methods such as the use of gunshot create physical changes to the body such as bleeding, which is typically managed by the client on their land. The veterinarian and attending staff may offer to clean the area should the client request it, especially when other horses will be in the area soon after. If the bullet exits the horse, it should be mentioned to the client that they may find it later. Waiting until the horse lowers its head will prevent this from happening. If the horse refuses to do so, it should be sedated before proceeding. This becomes especially important if the veterinarian is working with a large horse or is small in stature himself.

A properly executed gunshot will cause the horse to drop straight to the ground. Those in the area should be prepared for this. If the bullet does not penetrate the brainstem correctly, the horse may exhibit erratic movements, and therefore, another shot should be immediately taken. If the bullet does exit the back of the head, there will be two bleeding holes and likely to be more external bleeding.

### Captive bolt

Euthanasia with the penetrating captive bolt has many things in common with gunshot except for danger to observers. The captive bolt gun is powered by either gunpowder or compressed air and will extend the bolt 3 in. in toward the brain. The bolt must penetrate the skull of the horse and cause trauma to the brain, just like in any other species. The instrument is placed against the forehead of the horse using the imaginary "X." It may be advisable to sedate the horse as the captive bolt gun must be held perpendicular to the skull and touching the forehead for maximum penetration of the bolt. As with gunshot there will be a loud report and the horse will drop abruptly. The operator of the captive bolt must be positioned appropriately to prevent being struck by the falling patient. Bleeding from the nostrils is similar to euthanasia by firearm. Expected blood loss can be up to 500 mL. Extreme fracturing of the skull is very rare and should not be expected.

### Technical challenges

If the bolt gun is held at an angle to the skull, the bolt may glance off the bone and not penetrate. This is painful and not debilitating, so the horse does what would be expected and attempts an instant escape. He is now hurting, and afraid, and will be much harder to control. The horse may or may not go down, may or may not lose consciousness, and may run off bleeding. It all depends on the level of damage that has been done.

Captive bolt guns that are poorly maintained may misfire. If the gun cannot be cleaned and readied, another technique will have to be performed. This is never ideal for the horse or client.

For veterinarians who have never attempted this technique before, pre-euthanasia sedation is strongly encouraged. It is possible the bolt will penetrate, but not kill the horse. If the horse is already down, the procedure can be repeated, or in extreme situations, a pithing rod may be used to achieve death.

### Exsanguination

Exsanguination can be either internal or external and by itself, is already considered technically challenging. Internal exsanguination is usually accomplished by placing a sharp instrument into the rectum and transecting the terminal aorta. This allows the animal to bleed into the abdominal cavity. It cannot safely be carried out on an awake horse due to thrashing legs and would be viewed as inhumane. Death by exsanguination causes great agitation and fear for the few minutes when the brain is not receiving adequate blood supply. Even a horse in shock will respond to the cut and demonstrate great distress.

External exsanguination is usually accomplished by transaction of the jugular veins and the carotid arteries in the neck, similar to that in livestock. It is easiest to perform using a large, very sharp knife. Scalpels are often inadequate because the blade is too small and requires repeated cuts to be effective. The thick neck musculature and tissue also make it is easy to break a scalpel blade. External exsanguination is equally as stressful as the internal method in conscious horses and is considered unacceptable. Both are listed as adjunctive methods by the AVMA.

If the neck is not easily cut, more force will need to be applied to the blade and deeper cutting movements performed. This can be emotionally troubling for those performing it and any onlookers. Veterinarians are encouraged to practice this technique on deceased animals before attempting it with a client present.

### Special circumstances

Foals are generally considered easier to euthanize than an adult horse. However, their youth may make it more difficult to quiet them and keep them standing still for injection. Again, sedation may be used if necessary. Considerations for fetuses remain the same for horses as other mammalian species.

When injury necessitates euthanasia at a public event, heavy sedation or anesthesia may be used to quiet the horse until it can be removed and euthanized properly in private. Regular sedatives may also be given as long as handlers and onlookers remain safe. There may be instances when a physical method is required and the public should be informed as to why such means were necessary to prevent further suffering. Removal of the horse should be done as delicately as possible.

## Livestock

The method of euthanasia chosen for any individual case must be tailored to the client, animal, physical environment, and available resources. This section focuses on the three primary methods of euthanasia in livestock: (1) lethal injection by barbiturate overdose, (2) gunshot, and (3) captive bolt stunning. Where appropriate, other alternatives that may be indicated in certain circumstances will be presented for individual species.

### Inhalant agents

Inhalant agents for euthanasia of livestock is very rare, except in those circumstances where the animal is already exposed to anesthetic gases such as while undergoing a surgical procedure. The use of inhalant drugs to euthanize livestock is rarely, if ever, attempted due to the large volume of gas needed to euthanize a large animal and the availability of superior methods.

## Noninhalant pharmaceutical agents

### Intravenous injections
#### Cattle

Performed well, euthanasia by lethal injection is a very smooth procedure and is often considered the least aversive method of euthanasia for livestock. There seems to be common concern over difficult euthanasia where excitability, excessive agonal response, or a prolonged time to death is observed. These occurrences are often attributed to either poor venipuncture with a portion of the drug administered perivascularly, or severely compromised animals with compromised cardiovascular function. This is where the decision of whether or not to sedate an animal and whether or not to use a direct venipuncture or an IV catheter is critical. Above all, the most important aspect to a smooth euthanasia by IV injection of pentobarbital is rapid and complete injection of the drug intravenously. Using long (1.5-2 in.) large gauge (16-14 gauge) needles or catheters (3-5 in., 16-12 gauge) will aid in proper IV delivery.

Euthanasia solutions are most commonly administered intravenously in the jugular vein for cattle (Figure 5.54). The labeled dose for the drug is generally effective, although some individuals routinely increase this dose. For

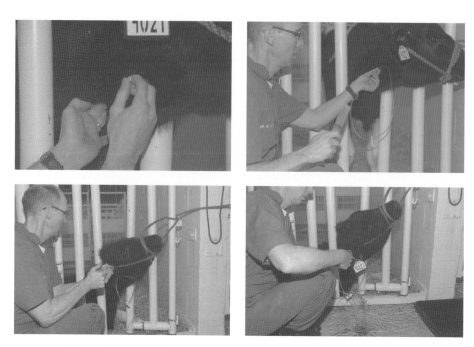

**Figure 5.54** Euthanasia of a calf by jugular intravenous (IV) injection. A 14-gauge 2-in. needle was used for the IV injection along with an extension set. The extension set is not necessary but does allow some freedom if the animal moves its head and neck while giving the injection. Note that when the animal becomes recumbent, it lays down to the side opposite the direction the head is turned.

sodium-pentobarbital-based euthanasia solutions, the labeled dose is 100 mg/kg. Most current pentobarbital-based euthanasia solutions contain 390 mg/ml sodium pentobarbital and the standard dose is approximately 1 mL per 4.5 kg (10 lb) body weight.

The jugular vein allows the best IV access for rapid administration of the euthanasia solution. Direct venipuncture or a jugular catheter may be used. It is recommended to use the largest gauge needle or catheter that is reasonable for the size of animal (18-14 gauge for calves, and 16-12 gauge for adult cattle). While the ear veins are an alternative, their size does not allow for as large a needle or catheter to administer the euthanasia solution as rapidly.

The animal should be restrained so that the jugular furrow is accessible for venipuncture or catheter placement (Figure 5.55). In both cases, the venipuncture is directed down the jugular vein with the flow of the blood. An extension set may be connected to the needle or the catheter to allow for easier administration of the euthanasia solution. It is appropriate to draw back on the syringe plunger after every one-quarter dose is administered to ensure that the needle is still in the vein. If not, the needle should be redirected or venipuncture should be attempted at another site. It is critical that the entire dose of euthanasia solution is administered intravenously and rapidly in order

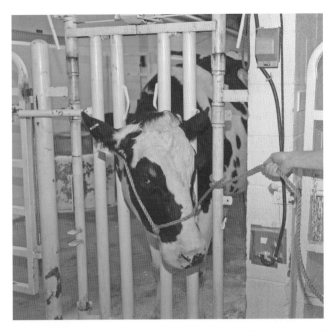

**Figure 5.55**  A head catch system with a solid wall and a swinging gate that can be used for physical restraint of cattle for euthanasia. Note how the head is restrained to the left of the animal. This will result in the animal most likely falling in right lateral recumbency upon euthanasia. This is important as it keeps the limbs toward the solid wall and allows safer access to the neck and jugular veins from the back or dorsum of the animal.

to have a smooth euthanasia with minimal complications. Many euthanasia procedures that result in adverse behavior or reactions in the animal are due to perivascular administration of some or all of the euthanasia solution.

To perform an IC injection, the location of the heart is identified either by auscultation or by palpation of the chest. The appropriate site for IC injection is generally in the 5th ICS at the level of the elbow or just above the elbow. A 3-in. needle is required for calves and a 5-in. needle is used in adult cattle.

Following completion of the injection, the animal will become laterally recumbent. If the animal was standing, it will generally collapse gradually over several seconds. Some paddling of the limbs may be observed. Once recumbent, it is recommended that the handlers and operator position themselves toward the backside of the animal to minimize the risk of being struck by the limbs. During this time, signs of unconsciousness can be assessed (Box 4.2). After respiration has stopped, the heart is ausculted to verify cardiac arrest.

Cardiac arrest can also be induced by lethal injection of a solution of KCl. This is considered an adjunctive euthanasia method and should never be used in a conscious animal. Once the animal is rendered unconscious by gunshot or captive bolt, a saturated solution of KCl is administered intravenously. The specifics of preparing saturated KCl were presented in Chapter 2. However, if some solid particles of salt are observed in the solution, then the solution is saturated at that temperature. A volume of 1 mL per 10 lb body weight is sufficient to induce cardiac arrest. The solution can be administered IV in the jugular vein. If the jugular vein is not accessible, then the KCl solution can be administered as an IC injection in unconscious animals.

Consideration of the disposal of the carcass is critical following euthanasia by lethal injection. The tissues of the carcass are potentially toxic to scavenging animals and the carcass must be disposed of properly. More details regarding this can be found in Chapter 6.

### Sheep and goats

As with cattle, euthanasia by lethal injection is performed with pentobarbital-containing euthanasia solutions. The standard dosage of 1 mL per 10 lb body weight is recommended. As with other species, it is critical that the euthanasia solution is injected rapidly and that it all enters the vascular space. Thus, performing a competent venipuncture or placing an IV catheter is critical for a smooth euthanasia. Clipping the animal's neck will aid in venipuncture (Figures 5.56-5.58). Most problems with rough euthanasia are due to either perivascular administration of some or all of the euthanasia solution or cardiovascular compromise in the animal. The use of sedatives prior to euthanasia may be associated with prolonged or rough euthanasia in small ruminants and may be due to slow drug distribution from hypotension caused by the animal's condition and the sedative.

Following administration of the euthanasia solution, the animal should calmly collapse into sternal, then lateral recumbency. The eyes generally remain open and fixed with dilated pupils. Corneal and palpebral reflexes are absent. Respiration becomes erratic and then ceases, followed by cardiac arrest. Once respiratory arrest has occurred, the animal should be assessed for cardiac arrest by auscultation of the heart.

### Swine

The challenge with performing euthanasia by lethal injection in swine is performing a successful venipuncture or IC injection. These procedures generally require suitable restraint. In debilitated or obtunded domestic pigs, successful venipuncture of an ear vein may allow for administration of euthanasia solution. Alternatively, venipuncture of the anterior vena cava, brachiocephalic vein, or jugular vein may be attempted in the neck. Because pigs generally resist physical restraint, this procedure will benefit from injectable sedation or anesthesia. Many pigs also tolerate being masked and anesthetized with isoflurane (Figure 5.59). Once the pig is sedated or anesthetized, venipuncture or IC injection can be done more successfully and with little distress to the pig.

Owners of pet pigs often request euthanasia by lethal injection over gunshot or captive bolt stun. In these cases, the owners often expect us to perform this in a way that will cause minimal distress in their pet during the procedure. This can often be done successfully by first anesthetizing the pig with an injectable anesthetic combination or masking the pig with isoflurane either

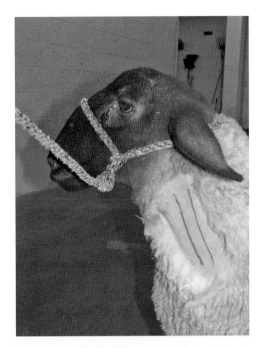

**Figure 5.56** Good visualization of the jugular vein in sheep. Shaving the neck is recommended for improved euthanasia by injection in sheep.

with or without sedation depending on the demeanor of the pig. Once the pig is anesthetized, a lethal injection of a pentobarbital-containing euthanasia solution (1 mL per 10 lb body weight) can be administered. IC injection is often easier than venipuncture. This method is well received by most pet pig owners.

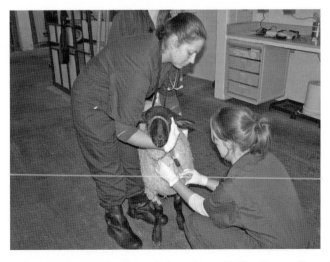

**Figure 5.57** Injecting the jugular vein in a sheep. Notice the gentle restraint and proper positioning used.

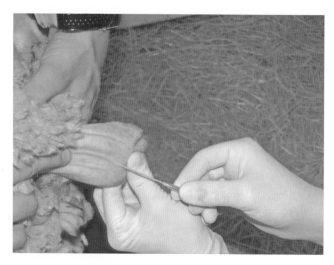

**Figure 5.58** Placing an intravenous catheter in the ear vein of a sheep.

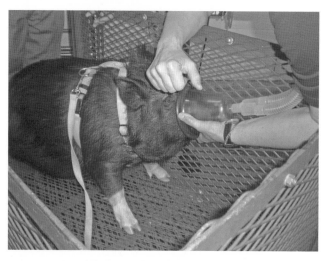

**Figure 5.59** This pig is being given anesthetic gas to prepare for an intracardiac injection of a euthanasia agent.

If this is a large domestic pig and cost is a concern, then a saturated solution of KCl could be used instead of the pentobarbital euthanasia solution since the pig is already anesthetized at the time of euthanasia.

### Llamas and alpacas
Euthanasia by lethal injection is probably the most common method used for llamas and alpacas. This method is less aversive to most owners and often provides a very peaceful death. The animal should be restrained physically, with or without sedation, or anesthetized. Some owners may request or prefer sedation prior to the euthanasia. Sedation should definitely be used if

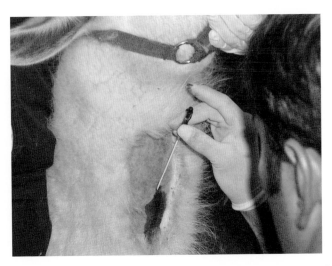

**Figure 5.60** Placing an intravenous catheter in the jugular of a standing alpaca. Note the obvious flow of blood. This should be minimized and contained whenever possible.

physical restraint is not adequate to allow for a proficient jugular venipuncture. However, sedation and anesthesia may prolong the time from administration of the euthanasia solution to cardiac and respiratory arrest. This should be communicated to the owner prior to the procedure so that they are aware.

Jugular venipuncture can be challenging in llamas and alpacas, particularly in intact males. Male camelids have thicker skin overlying the jugular furrow making it more difficult to identify the jugular vein and to insert a needle. Clipping the neck will aid in identification of the jugular vein. Initially clipping both left and right jugular furrows often makes it easier to appreciate the anatomy and gives more options should problems occur with the first attempt on one side. Jugular venipuncture can be performed standing, recumbent in the cushed position (sternal recumbency), or in lateral recumbency (Figure 5.60). When standing or cushed, it is best to hold the head relatively relaxed and level with the head slightly turned away from the side used for the venipuncture (i.e., if performing venipuncture in the right jugular, turn the head slightly to the left). Jugular venipuncture can also be performed with the animal in lateral recumbency if they will allow physical restraint in that position or if heavily sedated or anesthetized. When attempting to localize the jugular vein, it is often easier to see the jugular vein recede when you stop holding it off in the neck rather than watching for distension when it is held off, particularly if the animal is not clipped. Jugular IV catheters can also be used for both sedation and the euthanasia procedure.

If the animal is to be euthanized in a chute, then one must plan for extraction of the carcass. This is best accomplished if the side of the chute can be opened. Just prior to euthanasia, the latch for the side of the chute and for the head

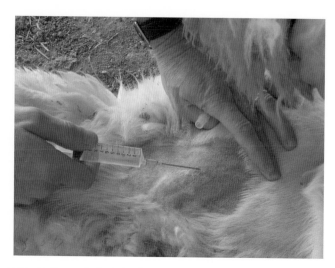

**Figure 5.61** Euthanasia by injection using the medial saphenous vein in an alpaca.

catch should be released to prevent these from jamming with the weight of the recumbent animal pressed against them.

The dosage of currently available pentobarbital euthanasia solutions is 1 mL per 10 lb body weight. The full dosage should be administered as rapidly as possible. This dosage is typically sufficient in most animals; however, there are individual animals that may require a higher dosage. Therefore, it is prudent to always have extra euthanasia solution on hand if needed.

IV injection by the jugular vein is preferred. This can be done either directly with a needle or from a catheter. The medial saphenous vein is an alternative site but requires that the animal is heavily sedated or anesthetized and is in lateral recumbency (Figure 5.61). If neither the jugular veins nor the lateral saphenous veins are accessible or suitable for IV injection, an IC injection can be performed. IC injection is most easily performed from the left side at the 5th ICS just behind the elbow.

Following injection of the euthanasia solution, the animal will gently collapse to lateral recumbency. The eyes will remain open and fixed, with dilated pupils. The corneal and palpebral reflex will be absent. Respiratory arrest followed by cardiac arrest generally occurs within 2-5 minutes. Some regurgitation, defecation, or urination may be observed.

### Technical challenges (Cattle, sheep, goats, swine, and camelids)
IV injections in these species have challenges similar to those in others. Vein visibility is one of the biggest challenges in sheep and camelids due to their thick layers of wool or hair. In swine, veins can be difficult to access due to their thick skin and fat content. When shears or clippers are unavailable and the jugular vein cannot be seen, a leg vein will have to be used. Sedation or anesthesia will render the animal immobile and allow for safer handling

while the legs are worked with. Typical leg veins to inject are the cephalic and lateral saphenous veins. If necessary, an IC injection may be attempted in the unconscious animal or a physical method used instead.

## Physical methods
### Gunshot
Performed appropriately, euthanasia by gunshot renders the animal immediately unconscious and is a humane method of euthanasia. There are significant safety considerations that must be acknowledged. In most cases of euthanasia by gunshot, the shot is made from a very close distance. This puts the operator at risk of injury from an animal that is not sufficiently restrained. In addition, there is the risk of misfiring the gun, either by accident or as a result of impact from a poorly restrained animal. There is the potential for ricochet off of the skull of the animal or from other solid objects if the bullet misses or fully penetrates the target. This increases the risk for personal injury or damage to physical property. The risk of personal injury and physical damage to property can be minimized by following these recommendations:

- Never euthanize an animal by gunshot indoors or in an enclosed space.
- Use the appropriate firearm and cartridge based on the animal's size and age (see Chapter 2).
- Be familiar with the firearm that is being used.
- Assure adequate physical or chemical restraint of the animal. Even a debilitated or sedated animal can suddenly lunge forward or to the side and impact the operator with the firearm, potentially causing direct injury or a misfire.
- Be familiar with the surroundings and consider what is behind and to the sides of the target.
- Any handlers assisting with animal restraint should remain behind the muzzle of the firearm.

While gunshot is more likely than captive bolt stunning to directly result in death, a secondary means of assuring death such as pithing, exsanguination, IV KCl, and pneumothorax should always be available if needed.

### Cattle
The animal must be sufficiently restrained in order to perform an accurate shot and maximize safety. The type of restraint is dependent on both physical facilities and the size and temperament of the animal. Physical restraint is generally sufficient for dairy cattle, docile beef cattle, or markedly compromised cattle. In these cases, a halter tied to a post may be sufficient. If the animal is recumbent, a halter may be used to tie the head back to the rear leg. The halter lead can be held freely by an assistant but it should be recognized that this increases the potential risk to the handler from either the animal or the gunshot.

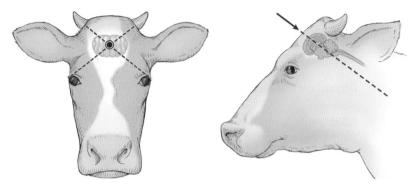

**Figure 5.62** The point of penetration for gunshot or captive bolt in cattle is at the intersection of imaginary lines drawn from the lateral canthus to the horns, or point on the head where horns would emerge. The angle should be either perpendicular or slightly angled to direct the penetration toward the brainstem and foramen magnum. (Image courtesy of Dr. J.K. Shearer, Procedures for Humane Euthanasia, Iowa State University Extension.)

In more excitable animals, a chute or head catch may be required for safe restraint. Using solid restraint equipment increases the risk of ricochet of a bullet that misses or fully penetrates the target. Chutes or head catches must have the ability to open on at least one side to allow for removal of the carcass following euthanasia. When using such a chute, it is very important to release the side *before* euthanizing the animal. If not, the pressure of the recumbent animal against the sides of the chute can make it very difficult or impossible to open the chute and remove the carcass. If this happens, it may require dismembering the carcass to remove it from the chute.

The choice of firearm and bullet was discussed in Chapter 2. For calves and cattle less than 24 months of age, a .22 caliber pistol or rifle with hollow point (young calves) or round nose bullets (juvenile and older cattle) are satisfactory. For adult cattle, a minimum of a .22 caliber magnum is required for consistent euthanasia. Shotguns ranging from 12 to 20 gauge loaded with slugs or No. 4, 5, or 6 birdshot will also work.

Humane euthanasia by gunshot requires proper positioning of the shot on the animal. The barrel of the gun should be within 2–12 in. of the impact site for pistols and rifles and within 1–2 m for the shotgun. The most common location for gunshot in cattle is at the intersection of two lines extending from the outside (lateral canthus) of the eyes to the base of the opposite horn or point where a horn would be located (Figure 5.62). The shot should be aimed either perpendicular to the skull or angled slightly up to direct penetration of the bullet toward the foramen magnum. A perpendicular shot has less risk of ricochet off of the skull but may only penetrate the rostral aspect of the cerebral cortex, resulting in unconsciousness but may not cause sufficient damage to the brainstem to result in rapid cardiac and respiratory arrest.

Note that this position is *above* the point of intersecting lines drawn from the eyes to the ears. A common error made by veterinarians with euthanasia

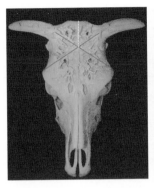 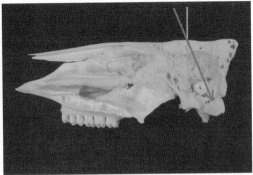

**Figure 5.63** The bovine skull showing the point of penetration for euthanasia by gunshot or captive bolt. In the lateral view, the difference in penetration of a perpendicular (white arrow) versus a slightly angled (gray arrow) shot can be seen. The angled shot has an increased risk or ricochet, but it will also cause more damage to the brainstem and vital control of cardiac and respiratory function. A perpendicular shot lower on the forehead may not even penetrate the cerebral cortex resulting in ineffective euthanasia. (Frontal skull image courtesy of Dr. J.K. Shearer, Procedures for Humane Euthanasia, Iowa State University Extension.)

by gunshot and captive bolt stun is placing the point of penetration too rostral or low on the forehead (refer to Figure 5.62). In some cases, this can result in completely missing the cerebral cortex and only penetrating the frontal sinus. When this occurs, the animal will generally lose consciousness, but may regain consciousness over time.

Alternative sites for gunshot in cattle have also been described. These may be considered when the positioning of the animal does not allow for easy access to the front of the head. The temporal shot is made from the side of the animal. The gun is directed horizontal and at a 90° angle to the side of the head at a point midway between the eye and the base of the ear. The poll shot is located from behind the head and the shot is directed from just caudal to the pole of the head aiming at the muzzle. Both of these alternatives have a higher risk of complete penetration of the bullet and ricochet and may be associated with a greater safety risk to bystanders (Figure 5.63).

In cases where the animal cannot be approached close enough for an accurate headshot, then a rifle or shotgun should be used. The point of aim is either the location of the temporal shot as described previously, the middle of the neck, or a chest shot aimed at the heart just caudal to the shoulder and elbow. Once the animal has fallen and it is safe, the animal should be approached for a head shot as previously described.

Following the gunshot, the animal should be assessed for unconsciousness and then confirmation of cardiac and respiratory arrest. The signs of unconsciousness have already been described in Chapter 4. The animal will immediately become laterally recumbent and lack a righting reflex. The eyes will remain open and be fixed, generally with dilated pupils. The animal will lack a palpebral and corneal reflex. Involuntary movement of the limbs may persist until after cardiac and respiratory arrest. These are not associated with pain or consciousness of the animal and the owner or bystanders should be forewarned of this prior to the euthanasia. These movements can sometimes be quite exaggerated and it is recommended for personal safety that the operator stay to the backside of the animal to assess cardiac and respiratory function.

Gunshot has a greater likelihood of resulting in cardiac and respiratory arrest and death of the animal compared to captive bolt because the projectile will continue to penetrate until it stops. However, a gunshot may not always cause direct trauma to the brainstem. Thus, it is recommended that a gunshot is still followed by a secondary method of causing cardiac and respiratory arrest such as exsanguination, pithing, or IV injection of saturated KCl.

## Captive bolt
### Cattle
Euthanasia with a captive bolt is similar to gunshot but has several advantages. The main advantages are a decreased risk of injury to bystanders or damage to property from a free projectile, and fewer regulatory considerations. The main disadvantage is the high upfront cost.

The choice of the type of captive bolt stunner was already discussed in Chapter 2. Some captive bolt stunners have different strength charges and the appropriate charge should be selected for the animal species and size that is to be euthanized. In cattle, the landmarks for captive bolt stunning are the same as for gunshot. The frontal site is generally recommended in most field and veterinary situations. However, in some cases, due to positioning and facilities, it may be safer and easier to obtain accurate placement from above and behind the animal aiming just behind the pole and toward the muzzle of the animal. The barrel of the captive bolt stunner should be held either directly against the animal or with a slight gap of no more than 1/2 in. The slight gap allows for a greater velocity of the bolt upon impact with the skull. In some models of captive bolt stunners, the bolt is actually recessed slightly into the chamber to provide an automatic gap and increase bolt velocity and higher energy on impact. This may improve penetration in adult livestock that have thick bone structure to the skull such as adult bulls and boars (Figure 5.64).

Because the captive bolt has limited penetration, it should not be relied on to always result in cardiac and respiratory arrest and death. For this reason, a secondary adjunctive method of inducing cardiac and respiratory arrest should always be employed such as exsanguination, pithing, IV injection of saturated KCl solution, or creating a pneumothorax.

## Gunshot or captive bolt
### Sheep and goats
Euthanasia by gunshot or captive bolt is an acceptable method of euthanasia in small ruminants. The equipment is essentially the same with appropriate choices for caliber of firearm and specific power cartridge used for the captive

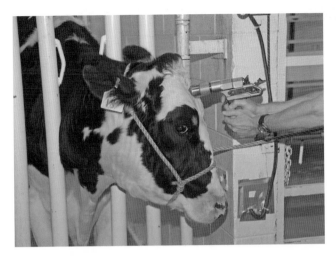

**Figure 5.64** Restraint and placement of a captive bolt stunner on an adult cow. Note the light restraint with a halter and that the head is turned slightly to the animal's left so that it will fall in right lateral recumbency, allowing safe access from the backside of the animal. The captive bolt stunner is placed directly against the animal for firing. Note in this case that the stunner is angled slightly from perpendicular so that the penetrating bolt is directed more toward the foramen magnum and the brainstem.

bolt stunner. A .22 caliber pistol or rifle is adequate for small ruminants. A hollow or soft point bullet is suitable for young animals and most adult small ruminants. The hollow or soft point bullet is less likely to penetrate all the way through the animal and thus has a decreased risk of human injury or property damage. However, in horned sheep or goats, particularly rams and bucks with thick skull bone structure, a solid point round nose long rifle shell is more suitable. Almost all commercial penetrating captive bolt stunners are acceptable for euthanasia of small ruminants.

Three sites are described for euthanasia of small ruminants, (1) the crown site, (2) the poll site, and (3) the frontal site. The crown position is the recommended method for polled sheep and goats (Figure 5.65). The location of this site is on midline at the highest point of the head between the ears, pointing straight down to the throat (Figures 5.66 and 5.67). However, in horned sheep or goats, the bone structure at the top of the skull may be too dense for optimum penetration. Also, this dense bone may increase the risk of ricochet when using gunshot. Therefore, the recommended site in horned sheep and goats is the poll position. The poll position is on midline just behind the bony ridge at the top of the head and aiming toward the muzzle or chin in goats and toward either the throat or the muzzle in sheep (Figures 5.68 and 5.69). It should be noted, however, that the poll site in sheep may result in reduced brain damage and subsequent recovery of brain activity over time. Thus, expedient exsanguination or other secondary method of inducing cardiac and respiratory arrest is recommended.

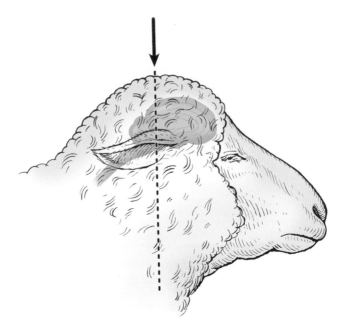

**Figure 5.65** Diagram showing both the frontal and poll sites for euthanasia by gunshot or captive bolt. The frontal site is suitable for polled animals but is less desirable in horned sheep and goats due to the high bone density in the front of the skull. (Image courtesy of Dr. J.K. Shearer, Procedures for Humane Euthanasia, Iowa State University Extension.)

The frontal position is described but is only recommended for polled sheep. This site is located on midline just above the eyes with the shot directed in line with the neck (Figure 5.70). The angle needed for a proper shot at this site increases the risk of ricochet with gunshot, particularly in horned animals (Figure 5.71). In goats, the brain is located more caudally, making this site less acceptable for goats than in sheep.

Following gunshot or captive bolt stun, the animal should become immediately recumbent and unconscious. Tonic seizure may be observed and may progress to paddling of the limbs. The eyes remain open and fixed, generally with dilated pupils. The corneal and palpebral reflex is absent. Respiration is erratic.

To ensure death, secondary methods of inducing cardiac and respiratory arrest should always be performed following gunshot or captive bolt stun. These include exsanguination, pithing, IV administration of a saturated KCl solution, or opening the chest to cause a pneumothorax. The methods for these procedures are the same as in cattle.

### Swine

Of all the livestock species, pigs are probably the most challenging animal to euthanize by gunshot or captive bolt. This is in part because of their cranial anatomy and also the difficulty to get sufficient restraint to allow for accurate placement of the shot. Pigs have a much more developed skull structure with

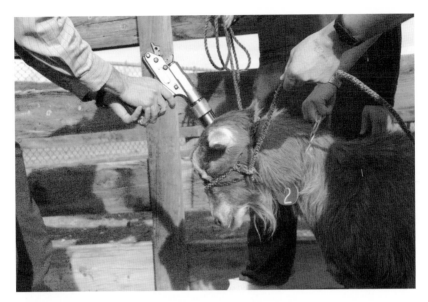

**Figure 5.66**  Euthanasia of a goat using a captive bolt gun in the crown position.

thick frontal bones and thick sinuses covering the brain. In addition, the target area is very small.

As with all species, proper selection of firearm or captive bolt stunner is critical. While a .22 caliber pistol or rifle may be adequate for young or juvenile pigs, larger caliber firearms are necessary for adult pigs, particularly boars. A minimum of a .22 magnum should be used on adult sows and a minimum of a .357 should be used on adult boars. Because of the heavy bone structure and sloped anatomy of the skull, solid point round nose bullets should be used to maximize penetration and minimize ricochet. An appropriate captive bolt stunner should have an elongated bolt to provide sufficient penetration through the frontal sinuses to the brain in adult swine.

Pigs, in general, are a difficult species to approach closely without confinement or restraint. This is necessary to allow for accurate placement of the firearm or captive bolt stunner. A nose snare may be used if necessary but will increase the distress in the animal. However, it may provide the opportunity for a more accurate shot and thus minimize the potential for pain and further distress in the animal. If a snare is used, the holder should stand behind the operator of the firearm or captive bolt. Alternatively, the animal may first be sedated to reduce movement and allow for a more accurate shot with less distress in the animal.

The frontal site is recommended for gunshot or captive bolt stunning in pigs. Placement of the gun or captive bolt is in the center of the forehead 1–2 cm above eye level (3–4 cm in larger sows and boars) aiming toward the foramen magnum and spinal canal (Figure 5.72). A transverse temporal shot (Figure 5.72) or an oblique shot (Figure 5.73) from behind the ear directed toward the

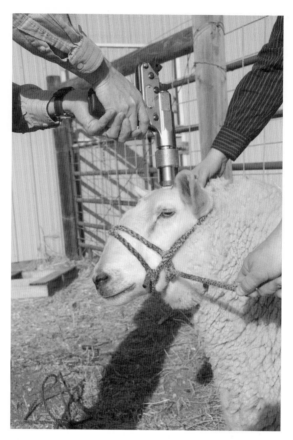

**Figure 5.67**   Euthanasia of a sheep using a captive bolt gun in the crown position.

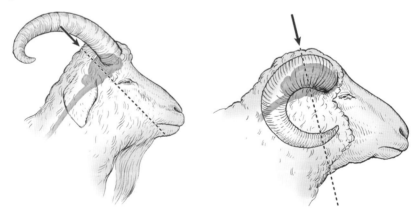

**Figure 5.68**   The poll site for gunshot or captive bolt stunning used in polled or horned sheep and goats. The point of entry is just behind the ridge line of the poll and thus slightly behind the crown site. In sheep, the aiming point is toward the throat. In goats, the aiming point is either toward the throat, like sheep, or the muzzle of the animal muzzle of the the animal. (Image courtesy of Dr. J.K. Shearer, Procedures for Humane Euthanasia, Iowa State University Extension.)

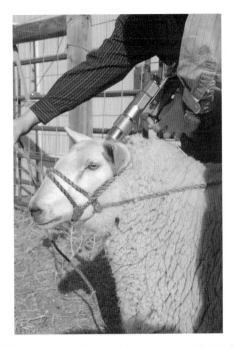

**Figure 5.69** Euthanasia of a sheep using a captive bolt gun in the poll position.

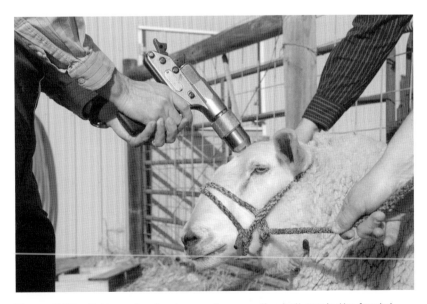

**Figure 5.70** Euthanasia of a sheep using a captive bolt gun in the frontal position.

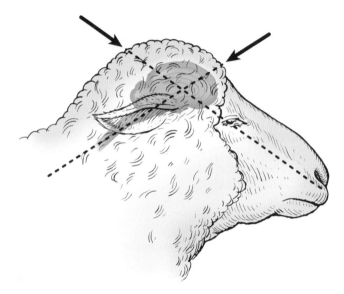

**Figure 5.71** Diagram showing the crown site for euthanasia with gunshot or captive bolt in sheep or goats. This site is acceptable for sheep and goats without horns but is considered less reliable in horned sheep and goats due to the more dense bone structure. (Image courtesy of Dr. J.K. Shearer, Procedures for Humane Euthanasia, Iowa State University Extension.)

opposite eye are alternative sites acceptable for gunshot, but not for captive bolt.

Following an appropriately placed shot, the pig will immediately collapse. They often show a period of violent tonic spasm followed by tonic-clonic seizure activity. If an animal does not demonstrate intense tonic spasm and instead has milder paddling or kicking movements, then it is likely that the

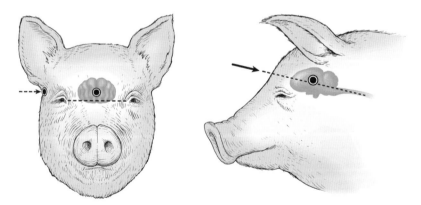

**Figure 5.72** Diagram of the sites for a frontal shot (acceptable for both gunshot and captive bolt) and the temporal shot (acceptable for gunshot only) in swine. (Image courtesy of Dr. J.K. Shearer, Procedures for Humane Euthanasia, Iowa State University Extension.)

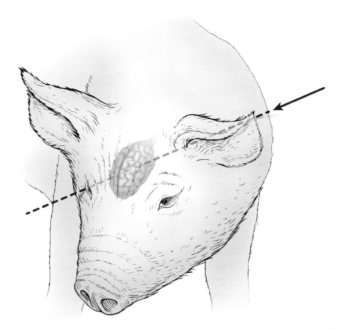

**Figure 5.73** Diagram showing the point of aim and direction for an oblique shot that can be used with a firearm for euthanasia of swine. (Image courtesy of Dr. J.K. Shearer, Procedures for Humane Euthanasia, Iowa State University Extension.)

stunning was ineffective and it should be repeated immediately. During this time, the animal should have open, fixed eyes with dilated pupils. The corneal reflex should be absent.

A secondary method of assuring cardiac and respiratory arrest should be performed as quickly as possible, ideally during the tonic phase and before the clonic phase. If employing exsanguination, a chest stick should be performed in order to sever the common carotid arteries and other major blood vessels near the heart.

### Llamas and alpacas
Gunshot or captive bolt stun is most easily performed with the animal standing or cushed. This allows the best access to the poll of the head and an accurate shot. If necessary, the head can be restrained with a halter and lead, or a rope halter. A single lead can be used or if more restraint is necessary, two leads can be used to hold the head steady to the left and the right. The leads should be tied off to a post or other sturdy object. Alternatively, the handlers holding the leads should be positioned to the side and behind the person performing the euthanasia to minimize risk of injury from a ricochet.

Euthanasia by gunshot or captive bolt is acceptable in llamas and alpacas, although not as commonly elected by owners. For gunshot, a .22 caliber hollow or soft point long rifle shell is adequate for alpacas and young llamas and a .22 caliber round nose long rifle shell is best for adult llamas. Most penetrating

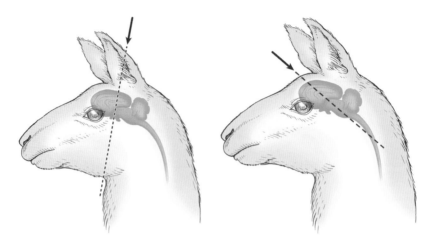

**Figure 5.74** Sites for gunshot or captive bolt stunning in llamas and alpacas. The crown site (left) is located at the top of the head on midline directly between the ears and directed toward the throat. The frontal site is just above the intersection of two lines drawn from the eyes to the opposite ear and directed toward the foremen magnum.

captive bolt stunners are adequate for both llamas and alpacas. If the captive bolt stunner has different size blanks, the same charge recommended for sheep should be suitable for llamas and alpacas.

Two different sites for gunshot and captive bolt stun have been recommended in llamas and alpacas (Figure 5.74). The crown site is located at the top point of the head directly between the ears on midline and aimed downward toward the throat. This is similar to that described for hornless sheep. The frontal site is located on the forehead at a point just above the intersection of a two imaginary lines drawn from the eyes to the opposite ears. The shot is directed toward the foramen magnum. Even though the illustration does not show it, a bullet from the gunshot method would ideally stay within the neck and not exit the body. Whenever possible, the animal should be given time to lower its head and provide the veterinarian with a perfectly positioned shot.

Following gunshot or captive bolt stun, the animal will immediately collapse to lateral recumbency. The eyes will remain open but become fixed with dilated pupils. The corneal and palpebral reflex will be absent. In all cases, a secondary means of assuring cardiac and respiratory arrest should be performed such as exsanguination, pithing, pneumothorax, or IV administration of a saturated KCl solution. The methods for this are identical to those described for cattle.

### Technical challenges (Cattle, sheep, goats, swine, and camelids)
Physical methods such as the use of gunshot and captive bolt create physical changes to the body similar to that of horses and other species. Because of

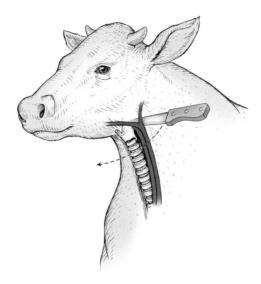

**Figure 5.75** Diagram showing the method for exsanguination by severing the blood vessels of the neck. A rigid knife at least 6 in. in length is inserted behind the jaw and just below the vertebrae. The cut is extended outward in order to sever the trachea, carotid arteries, and jugular veins. (Image courtesy of Dr. J.K. Shearer, Procedures for Humane Euthanasia, Iowa State University Extension.)

the thickened craniums typical to these species, especially those with horns, there will be more bone to penetrate. This leads to a greater risk of improper penetration by both the bullet and the bolt. An immediate second firing may be required to avoid pain and distress in the animal. As mentioned previously, a secondary adjunctive method may be required and should be readily available.

### Exsanguination

*Cattle, sheep, goats, swine, and camelids* Exsanguination, considered an adjunctive method by the AVMA, is performed by severing the major blood vessels of the neck. Once the animal has been rendered unconscious, a sturdy knife at least 6 in. in length is inserted behind the jaw and just below the vertebrae (Figure 5.75). The blade is then drawn forward, severing the trachea, carotid arteries, and jugular veins. An alternative method that is applicable to younger livestock is to sever the brachial vasculature. This is performed by lifting the forelimb and making a deep cut beneath the elbow to the shoulder (Figure 5.76). Again, this is considered an adjunctive acceptable method only when the animal is already unconscious. If the animal were awake and aware of the procedure, this would be considered a slaughter procedure, not euthanasia.

If the neck is not easily cut, more force will need to be applied to the blade and deeper cutting movements performed. This can be emotionally troubling

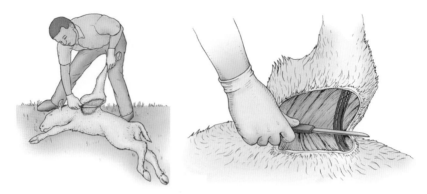

**Figure 5.76** Method for exsanguination by severing the brachial blood vessels. A deep cut is made in the axilla extending up to the shoulder. (Image courtesy of Dr. J.K. Shearer, Procedures for Humane Euthanasia, Iowa State University Extension.)

for those performing it and any onlookers. Veterinarians are encouraged to practice this technique on deceased animals before attempting it with a client present.

### *Pithing*

*Cattle, sheep, goats, swine, camelids* Pithing is another adjunctive method that can be used in unconscious animals. It is used to destroy brain tissue and cause death following techniques that may only render the animal unconscious, such as with a nonpenetrating captive bolt. Pithing is accomplished by inserting a rigid or semiflexible rod through the hole in the skull left by the penetrating bolt or gunshot. The rod is directed toward the brainstem. The rod is then moved in a vertical, horizontal, or circular motion to cause physical damage to the brainstem. The rod should be at least 6 in. long and can be made from a screwdriver or a Buhner needle. Disposable pithing rods are also available (www.pithingrods.com). It should be noted that pithing can contribute to the dissemination of brain particles to other tissues. Because of this and the risk of contaminating edible tissue with prions in BSE-infected animals, pithing is currently banned for slaughter animals in Europe.

### Special circumstances

Over the last decade, further consideration has been given to euthanasia of the pregnant dam and the potential for conscious distress perceived by the fetus. Current research suggests that the fetus is not sentient until after it has taken a breath (Mellor et al. 2005; Mellor and Diesch 2006; Mellor 2010). While the fetus will show reflex responses to stimuli in utero, there is no conscious perception of pain or discomfort. This has implications regarding euthanasia. First, in circumstances where a pregnant dam is euthanized, the fetus does not have recognition of pain or distress as long as it stays within the uterus until the time of death (cardiac and respiratory arrest). If the euthanized dam is to be prepared for custom slaughter, the fetus should remain within the uterus for a period of 15-20 minutes, or until dead.

These concepts also pertain to the ethical and moral considerations in dystocias where the fetus is alive but cannot be delivered vaginally and a cesarean section is not considered an option for medical reasons or by client request. These are very rare and difficult situations, the answer to which is very personal. However, the research indicates that the fetus will not consciously feel pain or distress if a fetotomy is performed on a live fetus that has not taken a breath. If this alternative is selected, the first cut should be made rapidly and result in severing major blood vessels (i.e., removal of the head for anterior presentation or a hind limb at the pelvis for a posterior presentation) allowing for exsanguination in utero. This method of euthanasia by fetotomy, while not a pleasant choice to have to make, should at least be considered physiologically humane based on current research.

Mass euthanasia in situations of exotic contagious disease outbreaks also poses unique considerations for livestock (Baker and Scrimgeour 1995). Human resources responding to a widespread exotic disease outbreak such as foot and mouth disease (FMD) may be limited. Also, the logistics of depopulating large numbers of animals on a premise with insufficient animal handling facilities must be considered (de Klerk 2002, Scudamore et al. 2002). Further consideration must be made for how the remains of the animals will be collected and disposed of. Euthanasia in situations of mass eradication of a contagious disease will be managed and monitored by federal and state regulatory health officials who will designate appropriate methods for euthanasia. If large numbers of animals must be euthanized expediently on the original premise, the most likely method will be gunshot. It should be noted that in the case of mass euthanasia, it is preferable to use a firearm that has sufficient muzzle energy to reliably result in death of the animal and not simply stunning the animal where adjunct methods are required. Firearms with a muzzle velocity of at least 300 ft lb are recommended for livestock less than 400 lb body weight. Firearms with a muzzle velocity of at least 1000 ft lb are recommended for animals greater than 400 lb body weight (US Department of Agriculture 2004, (AVMA euthanasia guideline review 2011)).

This section on livestock euthanasia techniques has focused on the three primary methods of euthanasia in livestock that are accepted by the AVMA: (1) euthanasia by lethal injection of a pentobarbital-containing euthanasia solution, (2) gunshot, and (3) captive bolt stunning. It must be acknowledged that unique circumstances can occur where the equipment required to perform one of these methods of euthanasia is not immediately available. Such situations challenge our ethical responsibility to follow established guidelines and our moral responsibility to relieve suffering. Morally, we face the consideration of whether prolonged suffering and natural death is preferable to a rapid death with the potential of additional acute pain and distress.

Methods of causing death in such situations should try as closely as possible to emulate the principles of euthanasia by rapidly rendering the animal unconscious, or at least in a state of very heavy sedation, followed by inducing cardiac and respiratory arrest. Small livestock (lambs, kid goats, crias, and perhaps calves) can be rendered unconscious by a very forceful blow to the head (see dog and cat techniques). This requires the use of a heavy, solid object that is forcefully propelled into the frontal area of the skull resulting in skull fracture and both concussive and physical damage to the brain. This procedure requires a high degree of force and accuracy to result in unconsciousness. The procedure is controversial, as it will not result in immediate unconsciousness when inappropriately applied. It must be followed by an adjunct method of inducing cardiac and respiratory arrest such as exsanguination, pneumothorax, or IV injection of KCl. Another alternative is heavy sedation with a drug such as xylazine followed by exsanguination or IV injection of KCl. This is distinguished from euthanasia of an anesthetized animal by injection of KCl in that heavy doses of xylazine do not render the animal unconscious prior to inducing cardiac and respiratory arrest. These procedures would only be considered justifiable in the uncommon situations where prolonged suffering and natural death by the animal was considered less humane than these alternatives.

## Unacceptable methods for domestic animals

There are numerous unacceptable methods of euthanasia, many of which were at one time considered acceptable until scientific study deemed them otherwise. It was decided that these methods could not reliably and consistently demonstrate the necessary criteria of today's euthanasia model, listed previously in the Introduction. An example of this is the once acceptable use of chloral hydrate in horses. Some techniques may be acceptable in some species and unacceptable in others. For a complete listing of these techniques, see the AVMA guidelines as mentioned in the bibliography of this book.

In general, the AVMA does not condone the use of injectable agents via the SQ, intramuscular, intrapulmonary, and intrathecal routes, with the exception of some injectable anesthetic agents such as ketamine or xylazine (only to be used in rodents with published studies on efficacy). The IP route should not be used in pregnant animals. Household chemicals, disinfectants, cleaning agents, and pesticides are not acceptable for administration as euthanasia agents under any circumstance. Other unacceptable approaches to euthanasia include hypothermia and drowning and any physical method in an awake animal that requires unconsciousness before proceeding. Paralytic immobilizing agents such as curare, succinylcholine, and strychnine are condemned as sole agents of euthanasia. They may only be used in an unconscious animal, but due to the availability of other agents, their use in general should rarely be needed.

When the attending veterinarian feels that euthanasia must occur for whatever the reason, any method of euthanasia is conditionally acceptable as long as the animal is pain free and death can be achieved as quickly as possible. If it is a client-owned animal, the client must agree to the terms of death and be informed of all possible outcomes.

## Death and associated signs

Signs of death are generally considered to be similar between all species. Body movements, reflexive breathing, urination or defecation, etc., commonly occur as the body and mind cease to function. It is important to recognize all signs of death for verification reasons and to prepare onlookers on what to expect.
Common physical responses to death in animals include the following:

- Body stretching
- Pupil dilation
- Urination
- Defecation
- Eye glazing
- Third eyelid extension
- Small spasms, that is, whisker movement, toe flexing
- Agonal breathing
- Borborygmi
- Thoracic air release, that is, airway sounds when the body is moved
- Opisthotonus
- Nasal fluid discharge
- Fly strike

Verification of death can be done by the following:

- Lack of pulse
- Absence of audible heart beat
- Graying of the mucous membranes
- Apnea
- Lack of reflexes, that is, corneal reflex
- Cardiac puncture; no movement
- Rigor mortis

The animal should always be evaluated fully to assure that death has occurred. Death is characterized by irreversible respiratory and cardiac arrest. The animal should be evaluated for absence of respiration for a period of at least 5 minutes. If the respiration is very shallow, it can be difficult to evaluate. An alternative is to hold a mirror near the nares and see if there is any condensation on the mirror indicating a breath. This works particularly well with livestock. Identifying a peripheral pulse can be difficult in large animals, so thoracic auscultation should be performed to confirm cardiac arrest. Alternatively, this could be assessed by electrocardiogram (ECG) or a doplar unit. Following death, the pupils will remain dilated and the eyes develop a glazed

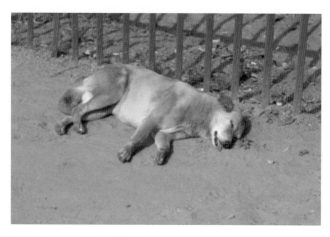

**Figure 5.77** Deceased dog with rigor mortis.

or glossy appearance. Rigor mortis, the stiffening of the body following death, will develop and may be appreciated as early as 10 minutes but may take up to several hours (Figure 5.77). It is critical that death is accurately confirmed following euthanasia. This remains especially important for those species that can dramatically slow their metabolism, such as reptiles and amphibians.

Of all of these signs, only rigor mortis indicates that irreversible death has occurred. Other signs can be seen during various stages of life, anesthesia, and near-death events with possible revival. A cardiac puncture test is commonly performed in shelter settings as another verification of death in small animals (Fakkema 2008). A needle and syringe are inserted within the heart to check for movement by cardiac muscle contractions. If blood is aspirated, and the syringe remains still, death is confirmed.

Urination and defecation should be expected with death in most animals. When appropriate, towels or plastic liners should be placed under the hind end of small animals to contain any releases. This is especially important if the pet is on a loved one's lap, within a family's home, or on any surface that will be difficult to clean. Urine can quickly saturate a towel, so another one should be within reach if needed. If heart or upper respiratory disease was present, something should be placed under the head to absorb nasal discharge such as blood and mucus.

Animals may exhibit very different signs of death depending on the method of euthanasia. The use of inhalants, injectable pharmaceutical agents, or physical methods all demonstrate fairly consistent physical changes depending on the species. The presence of pre-euthanasia sedation or anesthesia may also alter signs of death. It is commonly reported that animals in Stage 3 of anesthesia prior to euthanasia with a barbiturate exhibit less agonal breathing or body stretching (Cooney 2011). Animals given simple sedation prior to barbiturate euthanasia may move slower through all four stages of anesthesia and exhibit more involuntary signs.

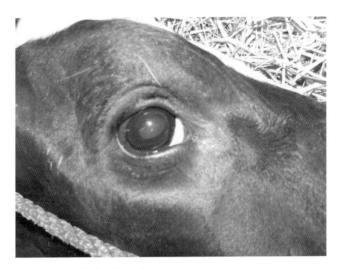

**Figure 5.78** Cow with fixed pupils.

Gunshot or captive bolt gun usage generally sets the animal up for a period of tetanic spasm that lasts for several seconds. The limbs initially flex and then gradually extend. This may be followed by hind limb movements that increase in frequency. In some cases, these may increase in force as well and can present a danger to the operator, handler, or bystanders. These movements are in part due to simple motor reflex responses of the extremities and are

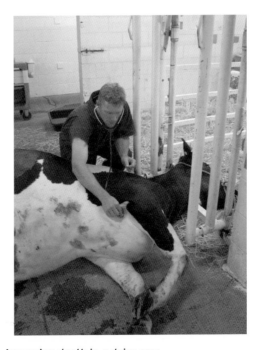

**Figure 5.79** Assessing death in a dairy cow.

exaggerated due to the loss of inhibitory control by the brain. It is important to be aware that exaggerated limb paddling may occur and explain to the client or bystanders that this is not an indication of consciousness. Immediately following gunshot or stunning, the corneal reflex will be absent and the pupil should become dilated with an absent pupillary light reflex (Figure 5.78). The respiration pattern will be slow and become erratic.

Depending on the effectiveness of the gunshot or the stun, respiration may cease and then cardiac arrest will ensue. Progression to respiratory and cardiac arrest is in part determined by the amount of damage to the brain and brain stem, particularly the medulla oblongata. Because of the free penetration of gunshot, damage to the brainstem is more consistent with gunshot than captive bolt stunning. However, the possibility of prolonged unconsciousness without respiratory and cardiac arrest, or regaining consciousness is possible with both methods. For this reason, applying a secondary method to ensure death immediately after the animal is unconscious is recommended for euthanasia with gunshot or captive bolt.

The species of animal being euthanized may also demonstrate particular death signs. Dogs, especially large breeds, may exhibit signs that are very obvious to onlookers. A good example of this is a large agonal breath with mouth opened wide and a loud gasping sound. Cats euthanized with barbiturates seem to pass a little quieter than dogs with little to no agonal breathing. Birds and reptiles tend to die with their eyes closed. Familiarity with the species and death itself will provide great insight into expected physical changes (Figure 5.79).

# Chapter 6
# Body Aftercare

**B**ody care options following the death of animals continues to grow in the United States. Depending a bit on geography, most owners have the choice of burial, cremation, rendering, or based on where they reside, body donation to a scientific institution. Unusual uses of the body, especially with livestock and horses, include donation to zoos for animal food, but only when euthanasia is carried out by means other than those that will leave tissue residue. Freeze-drying and taxidermy are also options for owners wishing to keep their pet looking in death the way it looked in life. The cost and options available are often determined by size and species of animal.

When an animal has been euthanized, whether it has been done in the hospital or external setting, preparations need to be made to ensure that the animal is handled according to the client's wishes. Whenever possible, details should be discussed prior to the procedure when client emotions are not as fragile and to expedite further steps. If they choose to keep a physical reminder of their animal, such as a clipping of hair, feather collection, or a clay paw print, these mementos must be prepared before the body undergoes any permanent change such as cremation.

Bodies should always be treated with the utmost respect, whether the client is present or not. Treating an animal's body kindly helps to lessen compassion fatigue (Figley and Roop 2006). Bodies should be moved in such a way as to convey this respect; using a stretcher to carry the body rather than dragging it is one example (Figure 6.1).

If the animal's body will be moved to an aftercare facility, it will first need to be prepared by the veterinary staff. Following confirmation of death and privacy for the family (if requested), the body should be placed in a containment setup of some sort for easier handling and to minimize contamination from bodily fluids, etc. Ice and other cooling systems can be used to keep small bodies cold until the client is ready for final aftercare. As of 2012 most veterinary services still use plastic bags of varying thickness to transport remains of small animals. A growing trend in the companion animal death-care industry is the use of pet caskets for transporting small animal remains to the aftercare facility, but this may not be financially feasible or requested for most pets

*Veterinary Euthanasia Techniques: A Practical Guide*, First Edition. Kathleen A. Cooney, Jolynn R. Chappell, Robert J. Callan and Bruce A. Connally.
© 2012 John Wiley & Sons, Inc. Published 2012 by John Wiley & Sons, Inc.

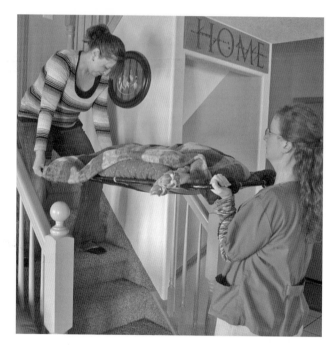

**Figure 6.1** Carrying a large dog down the stairs on a rigid stretcher.

today. Larger animals will require blankets or tarps to wrap or cover the body and are typically moved to facilities using livestock trailers.

When ready, aftercare facility staff will generally arrive to pick up deceased animals and transport them for burial or cremation. Most clients are not present for this transition time. If requested, arrangements can be made to have the animal picked up and taken immediately to the crematory or cemetery for burial. This minimizes the holding time and helps ensure that the client's wishes are carried out as quickly as possible. Some veterinary hospitals, or even the family, will bring the companion animal's body to the crematory or cemetery themselves to make sure it arrives in a timely fashion.

## Burial

Burial options include home burial, pet cemetery burial, or landfill internment. Animals of various sizes can be buried in boxes of various materials, in blankets, bags, or laid naturally underground with no wrapping at all. Pet cemeteries will have specific regulations for burials on their grounds. Landfill use is uncommon for family-owned pets, but is still available in parts of the country, especially for larger livestock. Disposal at landfills is more common for shelter pets, strays, etc., or for teaching institutions that cannot handle a large number of animals in their rendering facilities.

Veterinarians and their staff can help prepare client-owned pets for burial, regardless of their size. If the pet's eyes remain open following death, which

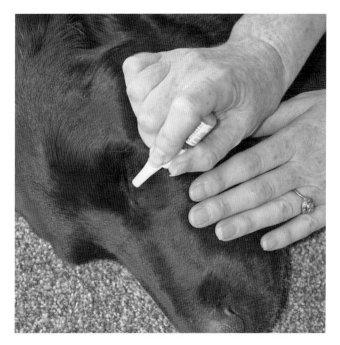

**Figure 6.2** Gluing a dog's eyes shut prior to burial.

is usually the case with mammals, they may be permanently closed using a liquid skin adhesive along the edge of the eyelid. Skin adhesives prevent the eyelids from opening and eliminate the risk of dirt/debris getting in the eyes during burial (Figure 6.2).

Any medical waste, such as catheters, tape, feeding tubes, etc., can be removed to return the animal to a natural state. Pets can be wrapped in special blankets or anything the family feels appropriate, including placing memorable articles such as toys, photos, feeding dishes, and collars/leashes/halters along with the body. When possible, the animal's body should be tucked into a position appropriate for burial before rigor mortis sets in.

If a client is considering burying their animal on their property, they must first contact local authorities to learn the rules and regulations of doing so. In general, every state, even county, will have specific guidelines that need to be followed to protect the environment and public at large. It can be difficult to get a concise, uniform answer as to how a burial should be done. All veterinarians should be educated on regulations within their state of practice to protect themselves from legal backlash should a client perform an improper burial. Clients should also be warned to avoid burying animals near trees with large root systems and be cognizant of utility lines that may be underground. Burial in the winter may not be possible in northern climates due to the difficulty in digging a hole in the frozen ground.

Scavenging by predators is a major concern when euthanasia is performed with an injectable agent like pentobarbital. Drug-laden tissue that is ingested poses a serious health risk, including death, for predators. Even smaller carcasses from dogs, cats, and exotics can pose a risk. A famous case of wildlife death occurred in 1999 in Colorado. Seven eagles were killed after ingesting pentobarbital-infused tissues from two mule carcasses. The rancher and veterinarian were fined $10,000 each (O'Rourke 2002). Many accidental poisonings of bald and golden eagles as well as other species have been reported (O'Rourke 2002; Krueger 2010). Several federal statutes including Migratory Bird Treaty Act and the Bald and Golden Eagle Protection Act may apply to protect these species.

Unfortunately, this is not an uncommon situation. If a veterinarian is found responsible for the accidental death of endangered species, such as one protected by the Endangered Species Act or the Environmental Protection Agency (EPA), the US government can issue fines up to as high as $250,000 per individual and $500,000 per organization, as well as imprisonment for up to 2 years. Because of this, it is imperative that veterinarians educate on proper burial guidelines, even having clients sign a legal document stating they understand the laws and regulations.

The Raptor Education Foundation based in Denver, Colorado, has created the National Euthanasia Registry to increase euthanasia-by-injection burial awareness. With registration, they provide a form to give to clients and keep on record should any legal action be taken against the veterinarian if a secondary wildlife death occurs. The goal is to protect all wildlife, regardless of the level of governmental protection. If incidents of wildlife death continue to be reported, it is possible that burial may not be allowed at all following the use of barbiturates.

Following are common animal burial guidelines often recommended throughout the United States:

- Maintain a 150-ft separation from wells and waterways.
- Maintain a 150-ft down gradient from ground water supply and a 5-ft separation above the ground water table.
- Bury the body with a minimum of 3-ft soil cover.
- Do not bury in a low-lying area, gully, or ditch that is prone to flooding.

## Composting

Composting is considered to be an effective means of recycling organic waste. It is a simple and easy procedure for the backyard gardener, but is much more challenging when the objective is to hasten decomposition of large animal carcasses. Approximately 6 months is required to completely compost an equine carcass (Brown 2007). The actual compost pile must be constructed and managed appropriately to be effective and to minimize contamination of the environment. A recently recognized problem with this means of carcass disposal is that pentobarbital used to euthanize animals may not be completely degraded by the composting process (Cottle et al. 2010).

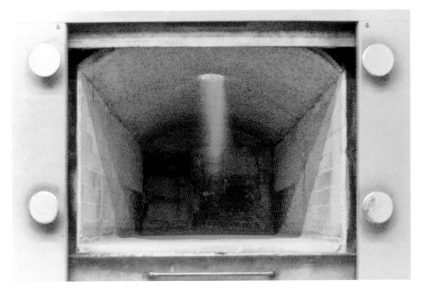

**Figure 6.3** Inside a crematory oven.

## Cremation/incineration

Cremation is the heating process that reduces animal remains to ash and bone fragments, followed by the processing that reduces bone fragments to minute, unidentifiable dimensions (PLPA 2009). According to the Pet Loss Professionals Alliance (PLPA), founded in 2009, there are three types of cremation offered for companion animals. Each is carried out within a designated animal crematory oven, but how the remains are handled is determined by the family or institution requesting the cremation (Figure 6.3):

(1) *Private cremation*: A cremation procedure during which only one animal's body is present in the cremation unit during the cremation process.
(2) *Partitioned cremation*: A cremation procedure during which more than one pet's body is present in the cremation unit and the cremated remains of specific pets are to be returned. Some commingling of ashes will occur, albeit reduced by larger separation spaces within the unit.
(3) *Communal cremation*: A cremation procedure where multiple animals are cremated together without any form of separation. These commingled remains are not returned to the owner.

As of 2011, there are no statistics indicating how many animals are cremated in the United States each year. Based on the increasing number of crematory businesses started annually, it is evident that clients are opting more and more for cremation over burial. It is generally less expensive than cemetery burial and offers more options such as scattering the remains, carrying portions within jewelry, or saving them until the time when they can be buried along with the client themselves. Cremation also ensures that any diseases or euthanasia solution within the deceased pet's body will not contaminate soil or another living being.

Legally, it is important that veterinarians learn about the crematory they are working with before providing referrals. Fraudulent acts by crematory owners in the past, using mass graves and deceiving pet owners with falsely labeled ashes, have led many people to harbor mistrust for the industry. Many practices today have an agency-type relationship with the local pet crematory. This means that an agreement is made with a particular crematory to send clients to them in exchange for financial compensation, special treatment for staff-owned pets, etc. If fraud should be discovered by a client, the veterinarian could be held accountable through vicarious liability for failing to exercise due care when referring clients (Hofmann and Wilson 2000). Veterinarians are encouraged to visit facilities, meet with staff members, and ask pertinent questions to gain a full appreciation of operations (Box 6.1).

We should mention that a new form of flame-less cremation, sometimes called Resomation, is gaining popularity in the United States and Europe. This process uses water and potassium hydroxide, or a similar combination product, under low or high pressure to degrade the animal's body down to bone fragments. It is also commonly called alkaline hydrolysis. This flame-less cremation is promoted as being more environmentally friendly than standard cremation and may become more popular in the near future.

## Rendering

Rendering companies are another option for body disposition in some areas. As of 2011, there are 205 rendering plants in the United States and Canada (NRA 2011). This option is relatively inexpensive, but is not an acceptable option for some clients. Veterinarians need to tell rendering truck operators if the animal was euthanized with drugs like barbiturates that are not inactivated by the rendering process. Barbiturates associated with euthanasia of horses and other species have been found as contaminants in pet foods (Myers 2011). Some renderers will not accept carcasses that were euthanized with pentobarbital for this reason.

## Species-specific considerations

### Dogs and cats

Dog and cat body care is much easier to manage than for larger animals, and due to the increasingly important part they have in family life, the aftercare options continue to become more personalized.

Pet funerals, casket use, and elaborate spreading of ashes are on the rise in the United States. Pet owners are treating beloved companions similar to

**Box 6.1** Taken from small business concerns: what veterinarians should know about pet cemeteries and crematoriums (*Source:* Used with permission from the AVMA)

- What kind of records does the facility keep?
- How long are the records retained?
- What type of system does the facility use to identify the body bags animals are received in?
- How will the facility handle multiple transfers from veterinary clinics to prevent loss of an individual body's identification tag?
- Are the bodies provided with toe tags or identification collars so that they can be identified even if they become displaced from the bags in which they are transported?
- Where and how are the bodies stored after receipt by the facility and before disposal?
- Does the facility have refrigeration and freezer capacity to accommodate the volume?
- What method is used to identify, store, and transport patient's individual ashes after cremation?
- If the facility provides for burials, what size plot is allocated for each animal?
- How many animals can be buried in a plot or grave?
- What is the daily capacity of crematorium furnaces?
- What is the breakdown between the number of communal cremations versus private cremations?
- How does the facility ensure that ashes of individually cremated pets are only those of the pet being cremated?
- What is the largest sized body that can be cremated on site?
- Can the facility handle large breed dogs or small farm animals?
- If communal cremations are provided, how many animals are cremated at one time?
- Are owners or veterinarians permitted to observe the cremation or burial?
- What is the standard turnaround time for receipt of a body from the veterinary practice to return of the ashes to the family?
- What kind of packaging is used for the ashes, and can owners open the containers and view the ashes?
- What type of fuel is used in the cremation?
- Do ashes contain chunks of bone or teeth, or are they sifted to remove those fragments before they are returned to the owners?
- Has the facility been inspected by the state, and if so, when was the last inspection?
- Are there any fenced-off portions of land in the cemetery area?
- What is the number of pets handled annually?
- Can the facility sustain its growth over the next 5–20 years?
- Does the facility engage in any business other than pet disposal? For instance, does it burn medical waste?
- Do the furnaces meet the EPA requirements for the location?

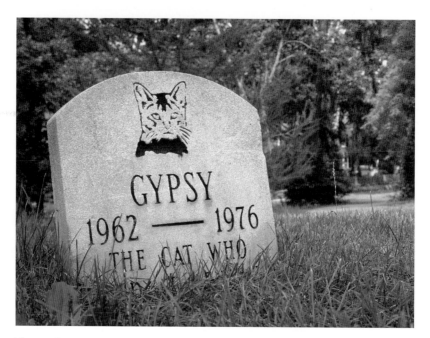

**Figure 6.4** An example of a pet cemetery grave marker.

human loved ones (Figure 6.4). Veterinarians are integral in the preparation for aftercare wishes and, by becoming educated themselves on all of the available options, can make the entire process easier for families. Within the rapidly growing specialty field of pet hospice, veterinarians and pet care professionals have an opportunity to partner earlier with families preparing for a loss.

If a dog and cat must remain on site following euthanasia, they should be wrapped in a towel, box, or bag to prevent fluid-release contamination, fly strike, etc. As discussed in Chapter 5, death changes the body very quickly and therefore, the pet and environment should be protected. Following death, bodies are placed in freezers kept on site at the hospital, shelter, crematory, etc. Cooling bodies is important to slow decomposition and maintain sanitary conditions at both the hospital and aftercare facility. Human mortuaries use refrigerated units rather than freezers to hold bodies, which may become the norm for pets. As mentioned before, physical mementoes may be offered to the family before body disposition occurs.

## Exotics

Exotic pets should be handled with the same reverence as other companion animals. For those clients wishing a private cremation, the ashes are returned in very small urns or decorative boxes. The client may have requested a paw print, a small group of hair or feathers, or the leg band.

Some species hold unique characteristics to consider when processing. A turtle shell, for example, will cremate completely away with nothing left to process. The large beaks of birds will also cremate and be ground down like the rest of the bones. Snail shells will cremate similar to bone. The smaller the body, the smaller the amount of ash will remain.

## Horses

Aftercare and disposal of the body is a major concern for the horse owner. These details should be in place before the euthanasia is performed if possible. Many states have laws requiring equine carcass disposition within 24–72 hours after euthanasia (Haskell and Ormond 2003). The equipment necessary to move the carcass would ideally be on site at the time of euthanasia. The body can be covered with tarps or plastic if there will be a significant interval between euthanasia and body disposal. Even a short time between euthanasia and disposition of the body may provide an opportunity for scavengers. A little time spent making these preparations can save much stress when euthanizing a horse. This becomes more difficult with an emergency euthanasia. Having a list of people or companies that will assist in carcass removal can be a greatly appreciated service for the horse owner.

In most cases, some form of equipment will be necessary to move the body. A tractor with a loader is most commonly used to lift the body. It is difficult to get large horses into some tractor loader buckets. Forklift teeth may be used to slide under the horse or chains may be wrapped around the legs and attached to the loader bucket. This is effective for moving the horse to a burial site or for loading on to a flatbed trailer or open truck. Tow trucks that have sliding beds for transporting disabled cars are also a good choice if the operators are amenable to this task.

Often, the horse owner will choose to load the horse into their horse trailer for transport. The tractor loader does not work well with a covered trailer, so a hand winch or many neighbors may be needed to slide the body into the trailer. It is possible to perform the euthanasia in the trailer, but the risk of injury to the veterinarian is greatly increased as there is no means of escape when the horse falls. Most rendering trucks have a winch system integrated into the truck to load the body. If the body needs to be transported on an open trailer, some form of cover will make the trip more esthetically acceptable.

Disposal of the body remains a significant problem for the equine owner (Meeker 2008; CDA 2010). In the United States, at least 200,000 equine carcasses must be disposed of each year (Messer 2008). If we assume the average horse weighs 1000 lb, this country produces 200 million lb of equine carcasses to be disposed of annually (Meeker 2008). Approximately one-third of these were sent to slaughter before 2007 when horse slaughter was banned in the United States. As this book is being written, some horses are still sent to Canada or Mexico to be processed for human consumption, but the vast majority must be cremated, buried, "chemically digested," composted, disposed of in landfills, or rendered (Meeker 2008).

Burying the horse would seem to be an easy option. While it is widely used in rural areas, burial has the potential to result in the greatest risk to human health and to the environment through ground- and surface-water contamination (Meeker 2008). Adding a layer of lime above and below the carcass may help speed the decomposition process (CDA 2010). It is critical that the horse is buried deep enough to preclude access to the carcass by scavengers, as the carcass remains toxic for extended periods of time. This was dramatically demonstrated when several dogs were poisoned after exposure to a horse carcass that had been euthanized with pentobarbital more than 2 years ago (Kaiser et al. 2010).

Because barbiturates are so persistent in the environment, most localities will not allow burial of horses euthanized with barbiturates in any area that might result in contamination of surface or ground water (CDA 2010). Burial in local landfills where procedures are in place to prevent water contamination is usually acceptable. Even if burial on private property is legal and unlikely to cause ground water contamination, it is advisable to use a utility locating service to be sure no underground lines are compromised.

There are certain situations, such as on large ranches, where the owner may choose to leave the body to natural disposition by scavengers. Potential contamination of surface water should be considered. The attraction of scavengers and flies as well as the odor produced are also important factors. In this case, drugs must not be used to euthanize the horse as these drugs persist in the body and can affect scavengers that feed on the carcass.

Options used for small animals such as cremation may be prohibitively expensive for some owners and may not be available in many communities. Some crematoriums may offer a head, heart, and hooves package as a symbolic cremation, which decreases the expense but does not address disposal of the carcass. Many cremation facilities are now equipped to cremate the entire horse, but the size necessitates it be quartered down first into a more manageable size.

## Livestock

Because of the variety of species and animal sizes, aftercare considerations in livestock encompass many of the same issues as small companion pets and horses. It is always important to discuss aftercare of the carcass remains with the client prior to euthanasia, as that may affect the choice of euthanasia method and location. Specifically, one must consider the location of euthanasia for large livestock to facilitate movement of the remains if needed. This could be to load the remains on to a trailer or truck for transport, move to a site for burial, or to move to a site for composting. As already mentioned, consideration must also be made to ensure protection of scavengers from consuming contaminated tissue if the animal was euthanized with a barbiturate-containing euthanasia solution. Lastly, the clients should be informed that there are fees for most of the methods of body disposal.

Small livestock may range in size from 10 lb (lambs, kids, and piglets) to several hundred pounds for calves, adult small ruminants, and alpacas. Remains for these animals can typically be placed in plastic bags or wrapped in blankets if needed for transport in a car or pickup. Larger livestock including adult llamas, swine, and cattle may weigh anywhere from 300 to 2800 lb. Movement of these animals generally requires mechanical assistance as with horses.

All of the disposal options previously discussed can be used for livestock. Cremation may be considered for pet livestock or livestock with other sentimental value. The charges for cremation are often based on the weight of the remains. Large-livestock owners may elect to have a partial cremation of specific body parts, often including the head and heart. Including additional bone dense tissues such as the limbs will increase the amount of ash returned to the owner.

Rendering is a common method of livestock carcass disposal, but over the last decade, this has become more expensive and is less available due to limitations and regulations placed on the rendering industry. The benefit of rendering is that the remains can be removed from the premises quickly and no further equipment or labor is required. The cost for rendering livestock varies by area from about $40 to $200 depending on the species and size of the animal. It is important to be aware of local rendering restrictions for livestock including whether they will accept animals euthanized with barbiturate-based euthanasia solutions. If a necropsy is performed on the animal prior to pick-up by the renderer, it is important to replace the viscera back into the carcass and suture the carcass closed with string or twine.

Many landfills will accept the remains of livestock. It is best to contact the local landfill to determine if there are any specific restrictions and what fees may be charged. Using the landfill generally has the benefit of a low-cost alternative if available but does require extra time, labor, and a means to transport the carcass.

In some cases, euthanized livestock are left in the open to be consumed by scavengers and decompose naturally. This method is generally discouraged as it has the highest risk for the spread of disease and contamination of the environment. It is considered unsightly by some and will have an associated odor as well as increased flies in the local area of the carcass. If this method is used, it is critical to determine this prior to performing the euthanasia so that an appropriate method of euthanasia such as gunshot or captive bolt stunning is used. Euthanasia by lethal injection of a barbiturate euthanasia solution would be inappropriate in these cases due to the risk of toxicity to scavenging animals.

Burial is another option for disposal of livestock. It would be rare for livestock owners to consider burial at a pet cemetery except in some instances for pet livestock. Burial on the premises is more common. Specific considerations are similar to horses. For large livestock, it requires mechanical assistance from a tractor to dig a hole of sufficient size and depth for proper burial. Owners may have the machinery to do this, or they may contract with a local excavator. While this is safer than leaving carcasses for surface scavengers and decomposition, there are still biosecurity and environmental risks. Local ordinances must be followed to protect against contamination of streams,

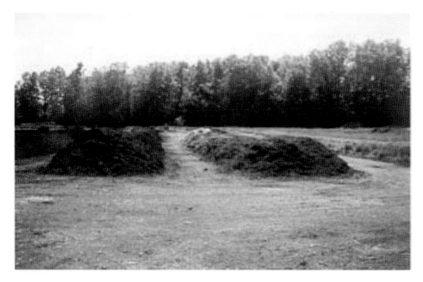

**Figure 6.5** Composting pile for livestock.

lakes, ponds, or ground water and wells. Specific information can often be obtained from local or regional public health department offices, the county commissioner's office, or the state department of agriculture, depending on the office jurisdiction in a given state.

Composting is probably utilized more for disposal of livestock remains than for any other species (Figure 6.5). The composting process has the benefits that it can decrease the pathogen load of the carcass, decrease odors associated with decay, can be performed any time of the year, is relatively inexpensive, and requires only a small amount of labor.

The basic procedure for carcass composting is to first establish a 24-in. bed of coarse, absorbent, organic material such as rough wood chips. This should contain pieces as large as 4-6 in. to improve aeration and drainage. The carcass is then placed on this bed and the rumen is punctured to allow for gas relief. Next, the carcass is covered with high-carbon material such as sawdust, dry stall bedding, old dry silage, or other coarse organic material. Including some semisolid manure will improve carcass degradation. There should be a perimeter of at least 24 in. of high-carbon organic material surrounding the bottom, sides, and top of the carcass. The composting pile is allowed to sit for 4-6 months. During this time, it is advised to periodically check the temperature of the pile at a depth of 6-8 in. Optimal temperature should be between 104 and 140°F. For optimum pathogen control, the temperature of the pile should be at least 135°F for at least 3 consecutive days.

After 4-6 months, the pile is checked to see if the carcass if fully degraded. If not, the time period can be extended or the pile can be turned to improve composting. The remaining composted material can be used for the bottom layer of a new composting pile, or used as fertilizer. Composted carcass material is appropriate for fertilization of trees, hay, or corn crops but is not recommended for low-growing crops for direct human consumption such as vegetable crops due to the potential of pathogen contamination.

A common problem with carcass composting is not using organic material that is coarse enough, resulting in poor air circulation. Another problem is too small of a pile, limiting heat retention and increasing external exposure. These problems can result in delayed composting, low pile temperatures, increased odors, and attraction of insects or scavengers. Overall, composting is an efficient and effective method of carcass disposal but does require some labor, resources, and a commitment to do it right.

# Conclusion

Euthanasia work, considered by most to be a less glamorous facet of veterinary medicine, needs further research within the techniques themselves to improve our understanding of methods. Scientific studies to fully appreciate current techniques and lay the foundation for new ones are needed in all species. Only through this can we fully appreciate when all the criteria for euthanasia have been met, the most important being the comfort of the animal. After all, it is they who are expecting a good death.

While the techniques and information within this book are broad and open for interpretation, it is the veterinarian working on behalf of the client and animal that will ultimately decide the best course of action. The decision to euthanize must be a collaborative effort, examining all logical possibilities and outcomes, for the benefit of the animal in question. We, the authors, recognize that not all decisions for euthanasia will be to alleviate suffering and hope that convenience euthanasias can be reduced through proper education of both the veterinarian themselves and the client faced with the decision to end life. Strong client communication skills will also go a long way to build trust and honesty when speaking on such emotional topics as this. Readers are encouraged to seek continuing education opportunities in the realm of client communication.

In the world of companion animals, a new emerging field of animal hospice is taking shape. The broad mission of animal hospice is to provide palliative care for the animal as it approaches death, either through euthanasia or the natural dying process, while also providing support for caretakers. Many of those helping to develop the role hospice care for animals recognize that euthanasia has its place and is deemed acceptable when the suffering of any species is eminent. For more information on animal hospice, contact the International Association of Animal Hospice and Palliative Care, www.iaahpc.org.

As we conclude this book, questions may still remain regarding mass depopulation techniques for animals. This is the rapid destruction of large numbers of animals in response to emergencies, such as the control of catastrophic infectious diseases or exigent situations caused by natural disasters (AVMA euthanasia guidelines draft review 2011). To address this area, the AVMA plans to release a new document, *AVMA Guidelines for the Mass Depopulation of*

*Veterinary Euthanasia Techniques: A Practical Guide*, First Edition. Kathleen A. Cooney, Jolynn R. Chappell, Robert J. Callan and Bruce A. Connally.
© 2012 John Wiley & Sons, Inc. Published 2012 by John Wiley & Sons, Inc.

*Animals*. Also soon to come are the recommendations on slaughter, the *AVMA Guidelines for Humane Slaughter*. Both of these documents will include many common themes in euthanasia work, but not all depopulation and slaughter methods meet the criteria for euthanasia and are therefore too broad for this book.

For those providing euthanasia, mass depopulation, or slaughter, compassion fatigue is a daily threat. Compassion fatigue is defined as exhaustion due to compassion stress, the demands of being empathetic and helpful to those who are suffering (Figley and Roop 2006). It can be theorized then that only people who feel compassion and empathy are capable of compassion fatigue. Another common term is the caring-killing paradox, used to describe the euthanasia-related strain among animal shelter workers (Reeve and Rogelberg 2005). Since veterinary medicine highly comprises people who love and wish to provide care for animals, a study conducted in 2004 by the Humane Society of the United States showed that one-third of veterinarians in practice are at high or extremely high risk of compassion fatigue (Figley and Roop 2006). Management of compassion fatigue requires commitment by the entire team of caregivers to provide ongoing professional training on the latest methods and materials available for euthanasia (Rogelberg 2007). Readers are encouraged to access their own risk at http://www.proqol.org/ProQol_Test.html.

# Bibliography

Adams CL, Bonnett BN, and Meek AH. 2000. Predictions of owner response to companion animal death in 177 clients from 14 practices in Ontario. *JAVMA* 217(9): 1303-1309.

American Association of Equine Practitioners. 2007. *Euthanasia Guidelines*.

AVMA. 2011. *Euthanasia Guideline Review*.

Baier J. (2006). Reptiles. In: C.K. Baer (Editor), Guidelines for Euthanasia of Non-domestic Animals, American Association of Zoo Veterinarians: Lawrence, USA, p. 42-45. ISBN: 0-689-70726-6.

Baker HJ and Scrimgeour HJ. 1995. Evaluation of methods for the euthanasia of cattle in a foreign animal disease outbreak. *Can Vet J* 36(3): 160-165.

Booth NH. 1988. Drug and chemical residues in the edible tissues of animals. In: Booth NH and McDonald LE, eds. *Veterinary Pharmacology and Therapeutics*, 6th edn, pp. 1149-1205. Ames: Iowa State University Press.

Brown LC. 2007. The effects of various co-composting materials on the decomposition of equine carcasses. Masters Thesis. West Texas A&M University, Canyon, TX.

Burns R. 1995. Considerations in the euthanasia of reptiles, amphibians, and fish. In: Proceedings: Joint Conference of the American Association of Zoo Veterinarians, Wildlife Disease Association, and American Association of Wildlife Veterinarians, August 12-17 (1995), East Lansing, Michigan, American Association of Zoo Veterinarians: p. 243-249.

Close B, Banister K, Baumans V, Bernoth EM, Bromage N, Bunyan J, Erhardt W, Flecknell P, Gregory N, Hackbarth H, Morton D, and Warwick C. 1997. Recommendations for euthanasia of experimental animals: part 2. DGXI of the European Commission. *Lab Anim* 31: 1-32.

Cohen S and Sawyer D. 1991. Suffering and euthanasia. *Probl Vet Med* 3(1): 101-109.

Cohen-Salter C and Folmer-Brown S. 2004. A model euthanasia workshop: one class's experience at Tufts University. *JAVMA* 31(1): 73-76.

Cooney KA. 2011. *In-home Pet Euthanasia Techniques: The Veterinarian's Guide to Helping Families and Their Pets Say Goodbye in the Comfort of Home*. Ebook. pp. 1-150.

Cooper JE, Euebank R, and Platt E. et al. 1989. Euthanasia of Amphibians and Reptiles. *Universities Federation for Animal Welfare*, Potters Bar: England.

Cooper JE, Ewebank R, and Platt E. 1984. Euthanasia of tortoises. *Vet Rec* 114: 635.

Cordes T. 2008. Commercial transportation of horses to slaughter in the United States: knowns and unknowns. *The Unwanted Horse Issue: What Now?* Forum . Washington, DC: USDA.

---

Cottle LM, Baker LA, Pipkin JL, Parker DB, DeOtte Jr, RE, and Auvermann BS. 2010. Sodium pentobarbital residues in compost piles containing carcasses of euthanized equines. *International Symposium on Air Quality & Manure Management for Agriculture* (September 13-16). St. Joseph, MI. CD-Rom Proceedings. ASABE. ASAE Pub #711P0510cd.

Daly CC and Whittington PE. 1986. Concussive methods of pre-slaughter stunning in sheep: effects of captive bolt stunning in the poll position on brain function. *Res Vet Sci* 41(3): 353-355.

Daly CC, Gregory NG, Wotton SB, and Whittington PE. 1986. Concussive methods of pre-slaughter stunning in sheep: assessment of brain function using cortical evoked responses. *Res Vet Sci* 41(3): 349-352.

de Klerk PF. 2002. Carcass disposal: lessons from The Netherlands after the foot and mouth disease outbreak of 2001. *Rev Sci Tech* 21(3): 789-796.

Dennis MB and Dong WK. 1988. Use of captive bolt as a method of euthanasia in larger laboratory species. *Lab Anim Sci* 38(4): 459-462.

European Food Safety Authority. 2004. Welfare aspects of the main systems of stunning and killing the main commercial species of animals. *The EFSA Journal* 24: 1-29.

Fakkema D. 2008. Euthanasia by injection–Training guide. *American Humane Association*, p. 29.

Figley CR and Roop RG. 2006. *Compassion Fatigue in the Animal Care Community*, p. 11. Washington, DC: Humane Society Press.

Flecknell PA, Roughan JV, and Hedenqvist P. 1999. Induction of anesthesia with sevoflurane and isoflurane in the rabbit. *Lab Anim Sci* 33(1): 41-46.

Grandin T. 1998. Objective scoring of animal handling and stunning practices in slaughter plants. *JAVMA* 212: 36-39.

Grier RL and Schaffer CB. 1990. Evaluation of intraperitoneal and intrahepatic administration of a euthanasia agent in animal shelter cats. *JAVMA* 197(12): 1611-1615.

Haskell SRR and Ormond CJ. 2003. Waste management: equine carcass disposal. *JAVMA* 223(1): 48-49.

Heleski CR. 2008. Ethical perspectives on the unwanted horse issue & the US Ban on equine slaughter. *The Unwanted Horse Issue: What Now?* Forum. Washington, DC: USDA.

Hofmann M and Wilson J. 2000. Small business concerns: What veterinarians should know about pet cemeteries and crematoriums. *JAVMA* 216(6): 844-847.

Kaiser AM, McFarland W, Siemion RS, and Raisbeck MF. 2010. Secondary pentobarbital poisoning in two dogs: a cautionary tale. *JVDI* 22(4): 632-634.

Lagoni L and Butler C. 1994. Facilitating companion animal death. *Comp Cont Educ Pract* 88: 35-41.

Lagoni L, Butler C, and Hetts S. 1994. *The Human-Animal Bond and Grief*, p. 194. Philadelphia: WB Saunders.

Lenz TR. 2004. An overview of acceptable euthanasia procedures, carcass disposal options, and equine slaughter legislation. *AAEP Proceedings* 191–195.

Longair JA, Finley GG, Laniel MA, et al. 1991. Guidelines for euthanasia of domestic animals by firearms. *Can Vet J* 32(12): 724-726.

Lumb W. 1974. Euthanasia by noninhalant pharmaceutical agents. *JAVMA* 165: 851-852.

Mader DR. (ed.). 1996. *Reptile Medicine & Surgery*, p. 278. Philadelphia: WB Saunders.

Mader, Douglas R. (ed.). 1996. *Reptile Medicine & Surgery, Mader, Douglas R.*, p. 278. Philadelphia: WB Saunders Co.

Martin F and Ruby K. 2004. Factors associated with client, staff, and student satisfaction regarding small animal euthanasia procedures at a veterinary teaching hospital. *JAVMA* 224(11): 1774-1779.

McCarthur S, Wilkinson R, and Meyer J. 2004. *Medicine and Surgery of Tortoises and Turtles*, p. 400. Ames: Blackwell Publishing.

McMillan F. 2001. Rethinking euthanasia: death as an unintentional outcome. *JAVMA* 219(9): 1204-1206.

Meeker DL. 2008. Panel: Unwanted horse issues; carcass disposal options. *The Unwanted Horse Issue: What Now?* Forum. Washington, DC: USDA.

Mellor DJ. 2010. Galloping colts, fetal feelings, and reassuring regulations: putting animal-welfare science into practice. *J Vet Med Educ* 37(1): 94-100.

Mellor DJ and Diesch TJ. 2006. Onset of sentience: the potential for suffering in fetal and newborn farm animals. *Appl Anim Behav Sci* 100: 48-57.

Mellor DJ, Diesch TJ, Gunn AJ, and Bennet L. 2005. The importance of 'awareness' for understanding fetal pain. *Brain Res Rev* 49(3): 455-471.

Messer NT. 2008. The historical perspectives of the unwanted horse. *The Unwanted Horse Issue: What Now?* Forum. Washington, DC: USDA.

Neiffer DL and Stamper, MA. 2009. Fish sedation, anesthesia, analgesia and euthanasia: considerations, methods & types of drugs. *ILAR Journal, National Academy of Sciences* 50(4): 357 (portions of this manuscript were published in Neiffer (2007), & Stamper (2007))

Pasquini C, Spurgeon T. 1992. *Anatomy of Domestic Animals*, 5th edn. Pilot Point: Sudz Publishing.

Plumb DC. 2005. *Plumb's Veterinary Drug Handbook*, 5th edn. Ames: Blackwell Publishing.

Pritchett K, Corrow D, Stockwell J, and Smith A. 2005. Euthanasia of neonatal mice with carbon dioxide. *Comp Med* 55(3): 275-281.

Ramsey EC and Wetzel RW. 1998. Comparison of five regimens for oral administration of medication to induce sedation in dogs prior to euthanasia. *JAVMA* 213: 240-242.

Reeve CL, Rogelberg SG, Spitzmüller C, and Digiacomo N. 2005. The caring-killing paradox: euthanasia-related strain among animal-shelter workers. *J Appl Soc Psychol* 35: 119-143.

Rhoades RH. 2002. *Euthanasia Training Manual*, pp. 1-151. Washington, DC: Humane Society of the United States.

Rogelberg SG, Reeve CL, Spitzmüller C, Clark O, Natalie DiGiacomo N, Schultz L, Walker A, Gill P, and Carter, N. 2007. Animal Shelter Worker Turnover: The Impact of Euthanasia Rates, Euthanasia Practices, and Human Resource Practices. *Journal of the American Veterinary Medical Association* 230: 713-719.

Rollin B. 2006. Euthanasia and quality of life. Commentary, *JAVMA* 228(7): 1014-1016.

Scudamore JM, Trevelyan GM, Tas MV, Varley EM, and Hickman GA. 2002. Carcass disposal: lessons from Great Britain following the foot and mouth disease outbreaks of 2001. *Rev Sci Tech* 21(3): 775-787.

Torreilles SL, McClure DE, and Green SL. 2009. Evaluation and refinement of euthanasia methods for *Xenopus laevis*. *J Am Assoc Lab Anim Sci* 48(6): 708.

Tranquilli W and Thurmon J. 2007. *Lumb and Jones Veterinary Anesthesia and Analgesia*, 4th edn, pp. 274-281. Ames: Blackwell Publishing.

Villalobos A and Kaplan L. 2007. *Canine and Feline Geriatric Oncology; Honoring the Human-animal Bond*, pp. 1-320. Ames: Blackwell Publishing.

Voss LJ, Sleigh JW, Barnard JP, et al. 2008. The howling cortex: seizures and general anesthetic drugs. *Anesth Analg* 107(5): 1689-1703.

Wadham JB. 1997. Intraperitoneal injection of sodium pentobarbitone as a method of euthanasia for rodents. *ANZCCART News* 10(4): 8.

Wolfelt A. 2004. *When Your Pet Dies: A Guide to Mourning, Remembering, and Healing*, pp. 1-76. Bishop: Companion Press.

Wright KM. 2001. Restraint techniques and euthanasia. In: Wright KM, Whitaker BR, (eds) *Amphibian Medicine and Captive Husbandry*, Krieger: Malabar FL.

## Web References

www.aabp.org/resources/euth.pdf - practical euthanasia of cattle.

www.aasv.org/aasv/documents/SwineEuthanasia.pdf - on-farm euthanasia of swine: recommendations for the producer.

www.AEMV.org - pain management in rabbits and rodents.

www.ahc.umn.edu/rar/euthanasia.html - University of Minnesota (UMN) 2009. Research Animal Resources, Board of Regents.

www.anapsid.org/euth.html - Barten 1994. Euthanasia of reptiles, Melissa Kaplan's herp care collection.

www.avma.org/onlnews/javma/jan02/s011502d.asp - O'Rourke 2002. Euthanized animals poisoning wildlife. Accessed November 2010.

www.biosecuritycenter.org/article/carcassdisposal - carcass disposal of livestock.

www.nwnyteam.org/Dairy/Natural%20RenderingFS.pdf - Natural Rendering: Composting Livestock Mortality and Butcher Waste.

www.colorado.gov/cs/Satellite?blobcol=urldata&blobheader=application%2Fpdf &blobkey=id&blobtable=MungoBlobs&blobwhere=1251663391356&ssbinary= true - Livestock carcass disposal. Colorado Department of Food and Agriculture (CDFA), Animal Industry Division, e-News, Fall 2010. Accessed November 1, 2010.

www.colostate.edu/dept/lar/Pain_Assessment.doc - pain assessment in laboratory animals.

www.creighton.edu/fileadmin/user/ResearchCompliance/IACUC/forms/ Euthanasia_Guidelines.htm - exotic euthanasia.

www.dem.ri.gov/topics/erp/nahems_euthanasia.pdf - US Department of Agriculture 2004. Governmental resource for euthanasia in livestock. National animal health emergency management system guidelines, operational guidelines, euthanasia.

www.efsa.europa.eu/en/scdocs/doc/45ax1.pdf - welfare aspects of animal stunning and killing methods.

www.fda.gov/AnimalVeterinary/NewsEvents/FDAVeterinarianNewsletter/ ucm093929.htm - Myers M. CVM Scientists develop PCR test to determine source of animal products in feed, pet food. FDA veterinarian newsletter 2004. Accessed February 2011.

www.fws.gov/southeast/news/2002/12-03sec poisoning fact sheet.pdf - Krueger BW and Krueger KA. Secondary pentobarbital poisoning of wildlife. US FWS fact sheet. Accessed November 2010.

www.icam-coalition.org/downloads/Methods%20for%20the%20euthanasia%20 of%20dogs%20and%20cats-%20English.pdf - world society for the protection of animals euthanasia document.

www.iccfa.com/groups/pet-loss-professionals-alliance - PLPA 2009. Definitions for cremation.

www.justice.gov/dea/index.htm – information on holding and dispensing controlled substances.

www.link.vet.ed.ac.uk/animalpain/ – animal pain.

www.nal.usda.gov/awic/newsletters/v11n3/11n3hany.htm – AWIC 2002. Guidelines for police officers when responding to emergency animal incidents.

www.nationalrenderers.org/about/process – NRA 2011. Rendering processes.

www.ncbi.nlm.nih.gov/pmc/articles/PMC2755021/ – amphibian euthanasia.

www.ocw.tufts.edu/Content/60/lecturenotes/799308 – exotic euthanasia.

www.omafra.gov.on.ca/english/livestock/horses/facts/info_euthanasia.pdf – Wright B, Rietveld G, and Kenney D. May 2009. Euthanasia of horses. Ontario Ministry of Agriculture and Food INFO Sheet. Accessed February 2011.

www.pork.org/filelibrary/Factsheets/Well-Being/CaptiveBolt.pdf – captive bolt euthanasia in pigs.

www.research.cornell.edu/care/documents/ACUPs/ACUP306.pdf – fish and amphibian euthanasia. Cornell University, Institutional Animal Care and Use Committee, ACUP 306.02. Original author/date: Brown C., April 17, 2003.

www.research.fiu.edu/compliance/animalCareFacility/sop/SOP%20302.01.pdf – exotic euthanasia.

www.research.uiowa.edu/animal/?get=euthanasia#general anesthesia – exotic euthanasia.

www.rwjms.umdnj.edu/research/orsp/ra/documents/04_Euthanasia_Policy_2006-1.pdf – exotic euthanasia.

www.theodora.com/rodent_laboratory/guideline_01_1.html

www.utexas.edu/research/rsc/iacuc/forms/guideline02.pdf – exotic euthanasia.

www.vdpam.iastate.edu/HumaneEuthanasia/pref.htm – euthanasia of livestock.

www.vet.ucr.edu/Primer/Biomethodology/Euthanasia.htm – exotic euthanasia.

www.vetmed.iastate.edu/HumaneEuthanasia – humane euthanasia.

www.vetmed.iastate.edu/sites/default/files/vdpam/Extension/Dairy/Programs/Humane%20Euthanasia/Download%20Files/EuthanasiaBrochure.pdf – euthanasia of livestock.

www.vetmed.ucdavis.edu/vetext/inf-an/inf-an_emergeuth-horses.html – emergency euthanasia of horses.

# Index

---

*Veterinary Euthanasia Techniques: A Practical Guide*, First Edition. Kathleen A. Cooney,
Jolynn R. Chappell, Robert J. Callan and Bruce A. Connally.
© 2012 John Wiley & Sons, Inc. Published 2012 by John Wiley & Sons, Inc.